Praises for This B
The Bragg Healthy

These are just a few of the thousa
receive yearly, praising The Bragg Health Books for the
rejuvenation benefits they reap – physically, mentally and
spiritually. We look forward to hearing from you also.

Thanks to ageless Bragg Health Books, they were our
introduction to healthy living. We are grateful to you and
your father. – Marilyn Diamond, Co-Author *Fit For Life*

The Bragg Healthy Lifestyle with Fasting has changed my
life! I lost weight and my energy levels went through the
roof. I look forward to "Fasting" days. I think better and I
am a better husband and father. Thank you Patricia, this
has been a great blessing in my life. Also, thank you for your
sharing the Bragg Healthy Lifestyle at our "AOL" Conference.
– Byron H. Elton, VP Entertainment, Time Warner AOL

Thank you Patricia for our first meeting in London in 1968.
When I was feeling my years, you gave me your *Miracle of
Fasting* Book – it got me exercising – doing brisk walking and
eating more wisely. You were a blessing God-sent and just
when I needed to get more healthily recharged for crusading.
– Reverend Billy Graham

When I was a young gymnastics coach at Stanford
University, Paul Bragg's words and example inspired me
to live a healthy lifestyle. I was 23 then; now I'm over
63, and my own health and fitness serves as a living
testimonial to Bragg's wisdom, carried on by Patricia, his
dedicated health crusading daughter. Thank You Both!
– Dan Millman, Author of "Way of the Peaceful Warrior"
www.danmillman.com

Bragg Super Power Breathing and Lifestyle makes the weak
strong and helps make athletes Olympic winning champions.
– Bob Anderson, famous stretching coach • *stretching.com*

*Just by paying attention to breathing, you can access new levels of
health and relaxation that will benefit every area of your life.*
– Deepak Chopra, M.D. • www.chopra.com

Paul Bragg saved my life at age 15 when I attended the Bragg Health Crusade in Oakland. I thank the Bragg Healthy Lifestyle for my long, healthy, active life spreading health and fitness. – Jack LaLanne, Thankful Bragg follower to 96½

Thanks to Paul Bragg and the Bragg Books, my years of asthma were cured in only one month with The Bragg Healthy Lifestyle Living and *The Miracle of Fasting*. – Paul Wenner, Gardenburger Creator • *gardenburger.com*

The Bragg Healthy Lifestyle and brisk walking (3x daily) for 20 minutes after meals, helped eliminate my diabetes! My whole body, circulation, feet and eyes have all improved. Thank you, may God continue to bless your Crusade. – John Risk, Santee, CA

As a youth I had a learning disability and was told I would never read, write or communicate normally. At 14 I dropped out of school and at 17 ended up in Hawaii surfing. My road to recovery led me to Paul Bragg who changed my life by giving me one simple affirmation to repeat: "I am a genius and I apply my wisdom." Paul Bragg inspired me to go back to school and get my education and from there miracles happened. I have authored 54 training programs and 14 books and love to crusade around the world thanks to Paul Bragg. – Dr. John Demartini, Dynamic Crusader, Star in "The Secret" • *drdemartini.com*

I had the opportunity to sit next to Patricia on a flight from Dallas to Los Angeles. Her honesty about my weight and health really inspired me to make a life change. One year later, I am 85 lbs. lighter and heart rate cut almost in half. Patricia you helped save my life! – Mike Ableman, Texas

Our great-grandmother will turn 100 in two weeks. She still kayaks, gardens, and shovels her own snow covered driveway. For over 80 years, she had one recipe for life: 2 Tbsps Bragg ACV and 1 tsp of honey mixed into water. This is the secret, she says, to a life worth living. Five generations of our family will celebrate her 100th birthday with Bragg's Vinegar Drinks! – The Alvina Sharp Family, Chanhassen, Minnesota

Praises for This Book and The Bragg Healthy Lifestyle

Your dad, Dr. Paul Bragg IS the FATHER of the natural health industry and the entire natural health movement. Everything that has been done in natural health and physical culture since has been based on the pioneering vision and principles articulated by Dr. Bragg. He gave us all our direction! – Dr. William Wong • *www.braggzyme.com*

I love Bragg Books and *The Miracle of Fasting*. They are so popular and loved in Russia and Ukraine. I give thanks for my health and super energy. I just won the famous Honolulu Marathon with the all-time women's record! – Lyubov Morgunova, Champion Runner, Moscow, Russia

---

I have known the Bragg Books for over 25 years. They are a blessing to me and my family and to all who read them to help make this a healthier world. – Pastor Mike Macintosh, Horizon Christian Fellowship, San Diego, CA

I've been reading Bragg Books since high school. I'm thankful for the healthy lifestyle and admire their health crusading to make this a healthier world! – Steve Jobs, Creator & CEO – Apple Computer/iPods

---

Thanks to Bragg *Miracle of Fasting* and *Healthy Lifestyle,* we are healthy, fit and singing better and staying younger than ever! – The Beach Boys • *www.beachboysfanclub.com*

In 1975 I was diagnosed with coronary heart disease. I followed the Free Bragg Exercise Classes and Lectures at Fort DeRussy lawn, Waikiki Beach, 6 days a week. 31 years have passed, now 84 years young thanks to The Bragg Healthy Lifestyle. In 1932 my father had severe hip arthritis and was hardly able to walk. He followed the Bragg Healthy Lifestyle, also had the Vinegar Drink and he cured his arthritis. – Helen Risk, RN, Hawaii

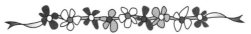

Improper breathing is a common cause of ill health. Changing your breathing patterns can affect and improve you mentally, emotionally and physically. – Andrew Weil, M.D. • www.drweil.com

c

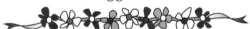

BRAGG PHOTO GALLERY

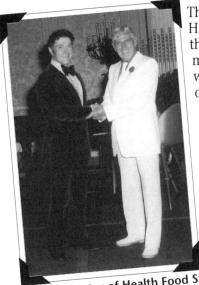

Thanks for The Bragg Healthy Lifestyle that you shared with me and are sharing with millions of others world-wide.

– John Gray, Ph.D., Author

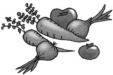

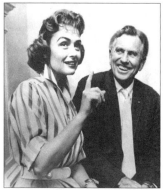

Actress Donna Reed saying "Health First" with Paul Bragg

Paul Bragg, Creator of Health Food Stores, with his prize student Jack LaLanne, who thanks Bragg for saving his life at 15.

PAUL C. BRAGG, ND, PhD.
Life Extension Specialist and Originator of Health Food Stores

In Medical School I read Dr. Bragg's Health Books, they changed my way of thinking & the path of my life. I founded Omega Institute. – Stephan Rechtschaffen, M.D., famous since 1977 • *www.eomega.org*

I've been reading Bragg Books since high school. I'm thankful for the healthy lifestyle and admire their health crusading for a healthier world. – Steve Jobs, Creator & CEO – Apple Computer

Paul Bragg with Actress Gloria Swanson who became a Bragg devotee when 18. Gloria often health crusaded with Bragg.

I'd like to thank you for teaching me how to take control of my health! I lost 55 pounds and I feel "great"! Bragg books have showed me vitality, happiness and being close to Mother Nature. You both are real "Crusaders for Health for the World". Thanks. – Leonard Amato

I lost 102 lbs. with Bragg Apple Cider Vinegar and The Bragg Healthy Lifestyle and have kept it off for over 15 years, staying away from white flour, sugar and other processed foods. – Dee McCaffrey, Chemist & Diet Counselor, Tempe, Arizona

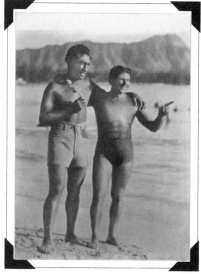

Paul Bragg with Duke Kahanamoku, the Olympic swimmer who taught Paul how to surf. His beautiful wife Nadine was Patricia's godmother.

e

PHOTO GALLERY

You have recharged me with hope, love and encouragement, which poured from your words. I am now able to fast. You have certainly improved my life!
– Marie Furia, NJ

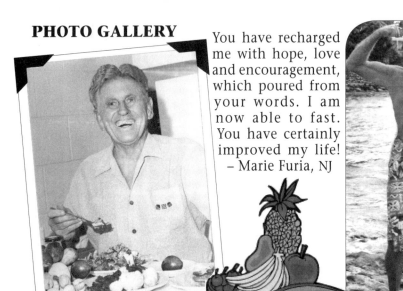

PAUL BRAGG STAYING HEALTHY & FIT!

Paul Bragg in Tahiti in 1925 gathering tropical papaya fruit.

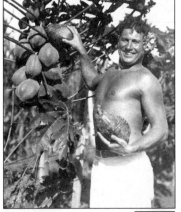

Paul Bragg owes his powerful body and superb health to living exclusively on live, vital, healthy, organic rich foods.

Paul C. Bragg and daughter Patricia were my early guiding inspiration to my health education and health career.
– Jeffrey Bland, Ph.D., Famous Food Scientist

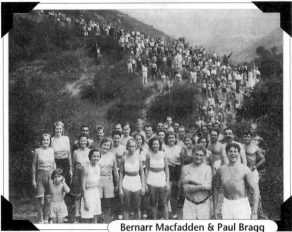

Bernarr Macfadden & Paul Bragg

A thousand happy Bragg Health Students enjoy hiking, exercise and fresh air on the trail to Mount Hollywood (above Griffith Observatory) in beautiful California, summer of 1932.

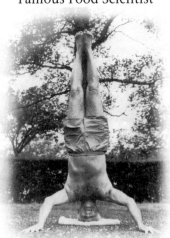

Paul C. Bragg
Regent's Park,
London, England

PHOTO GALLERY

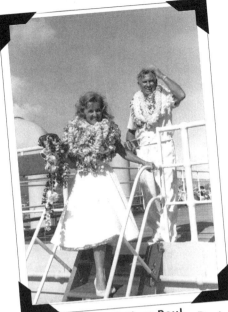

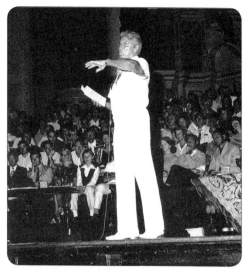

PAUL & PATRICIA BRAGG HEALTH CRUSADING

Patricia and father Paul leaving Hawaii for Tahiti and world trip in 1956.

During the 40-plus years Patricia worked with her father, she was right there beside him, assisting him on the Bragg Health Crusades world-wide. They were a team, when you looked at them, you would see only two people headed in the same direction.

Our lives have completely turned around! Our family is feeling so very healthy, we must tell you about it.– Gene & Joan Zollner, parents of 11, Washington

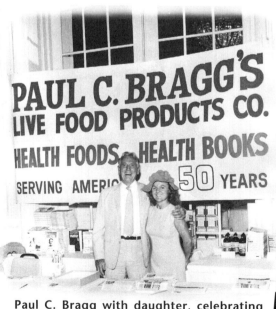

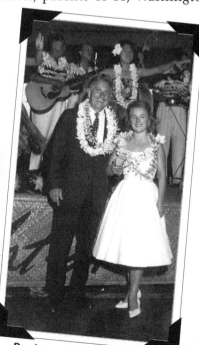

Paul C. Bragg with daughter, celebrating here over 50 years of Bragg Health Products, Books & Crusading world-wide, spreading Health around the world. *Time flies – soon will be 100 years!* –PB

Paul & daughter Patricia, Royal Hawaiian, Honolulu

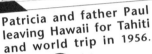

g

PHOTO GALLERY

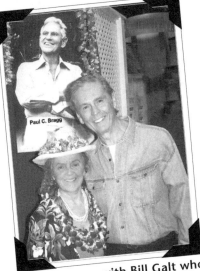

Patricia Bragg with Bill Galt who was inspired by Bragg Books and founded Good Earth Restaurants.

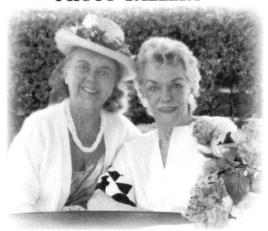

Patricia Bragg with Actress Jane Russell. Hollywood Star of the 40's and 50's and the favorite pinup of WWII. She starred in: *Paleface* with Bob Hope, *The Tall Men* with Clark Gable and *Gentlemen Prefer Blondes* with Marilyn Monroe.

Jack LaLanne with Patricia Bragg

PATRICIA BRAGG CONTINUING THE HEALTH CRUSADE!

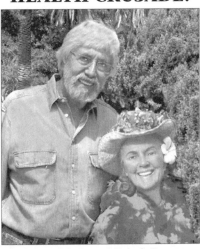

Patricia with Jean-Michel Cousteau Ocean Explorer & Environmentalist

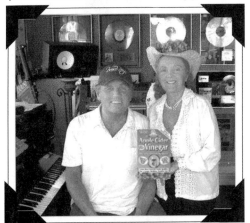

Patricia Bragg in studio with famous Beach Boy Bruce Johnson, Bragg follower for over 30 years. He played for her their latest records.

Dear Friends – you cannot know how greatly you have already impacted my life and some of my friends! We love your Bragg Health Books, teachings and products and are now living healthier, happier lives. Thanks! – Winnie Brown, Arizona

h

PHOTO GALLERY

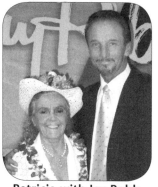

Patricia with Jay Robb

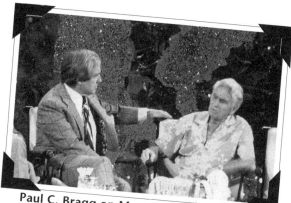

Paul C. Bragg on Merv Griffin Show, 1976

Paul Bragg inspired me many years ago with the *Miracle of Fasting* and with his philosophy on health. His daughter Patricia is a testament to the ageless value of living the Bragg Healthy Lifestyle. – Jay Robb, author of *The Fruit Flush*

PATRICIA & PAUL BRAGG NUTRITIONISTS TO THE HOLLYWOOD STARS

The amazing Duggar Family – "19 Kids and Counting" (on TLC) are big Bragg Fans. Their family relationship is based on respect, love, and Christian family values! Read their new book on *amazon.com: A Love That Multiplies.* We are thrilled the Duggar family loves Bragg Liquid Aminos & Apple Cider Vinegar.

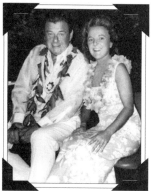

Arthur Godfrey with Patricia celebrating his birthday

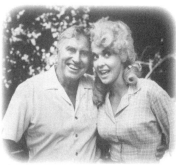

Paul Bragg and Donna Douglas, Hollywood's most beautiful, talented and best Health Girl. She played the part of "Elly-May" in the Beverly Hillbillies, which became one of the longest-running series in television history and was the #1 show in America in its first 2 years.

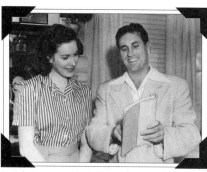

Paul Bragg with Maureen O'Hara, Irish film actress and singer. She was best noted for *Miracle on 34th Street, Rio Grande* and *The Quiet Man.*

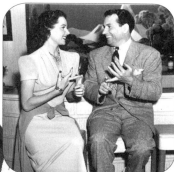

Paul with Actress Jane Wyatt, Emmy Award-winning American actress. She is best remembered for her roles in the 1937 film, *Lost Horizon* and the popular TV series *Father Knows Best.*

i

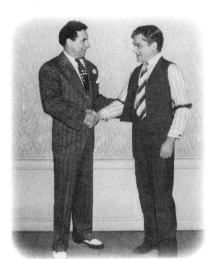

Paul Bragg with James Cagney, American film actor. He won major awards for a wide variety of roles. The American Film Institute ranked him 8th among the Greatest Male Stars of All Time.

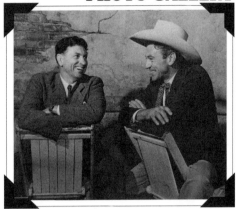

Paul C. Bragg with Gary Cooper, famous American film actor, best known for his many Western films.

Famous Hollywood Actress Cloris Leachman, who sparkles with health, says, "Bragg Fasting is simply wonderful. It is my solution to many problems. It is a miracle cure for sure . . . it cured my asthma." I praise Paul and Patricia Bragg daily for their Health Crusading!

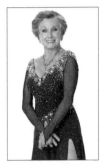

Cloris Leachman on Dancing with the Stars Show

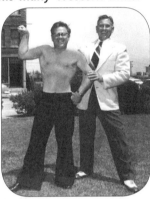

Paul with Mickey Rooney, American film actor and entertainer. He has won multiple awards and has had one of the longest careers of any actor!

I love the Bragg Health Products! My family uses the Bragg Liquid Aminos spray, even on popcorn for tasty treat. I recommend it in many recipes in my books.
– Marilu Henner, Actress & Health Book Author
www.marilu.com

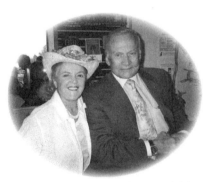

Patricia with Astronaut Buzz Aldrin, celebrating over 40 years since pilot of Apollo 11 first landed on the moon.

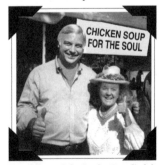

Patricia with Jack Canfield, Bragg follower, Motivational Speaker and Co-Producer of *Chicken Soup for the Soul* Series

I am a big fan of Paul Bragg. I fast and use the Bragg Aminos daily on my food. I even take it with me when I travel for my seminars, I wouldn't be without it! The world and I are blessed with the health teachings of Paul & Patricia Bragg! – Anthony "Tony" Robbins

BRAGG

Build Powerful
Nerve Force

A Cure For Those Dull, Dragged-Out, Hopeless, Helpless Feelings!

PAUL C. BRAGG, N.D., Ph.D.
LIFE EXTENSION SPECIALIST
and
PATRICIA BRAGG, N.D., Ph.D.
HEALTH CRUSADER & LIFESTYLE EDUCATOR

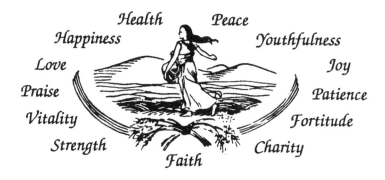

Health Peace
Happiness Youthfulness
Love Joy
Praise Patience
Vitality Fortitude
Strength Charity
Faith

JOIN
Bragg Health Crusades for a 100% Healthy World for All!

HEALTH SCIENCE
Box 7, Santa Barbara, California 93102 USA

World Wide Web: www.bragg.com

BRAGG
Build Powerful
NERVE FORCE
A Cure for those Dull, Dragged-Out, Hopeless, Helpless Feelings!

PAUL C. BRAGG, N.D., Ph.D.
LIFE EXTENSION SPECIALIST

and

PATRICIA BRAGG, N.D., Ph.D.
HEALTH CRUSADER & LIFESTYLE EDUCATOR

Health Science, Box 7, Santa Barbara, California 93102
Telephone (805) 968-1020, FAX (805) 968-1001
e-mail address: braggbooks@bragg.com

Quantity Purchases: Companies, Professional Groups, Churches, Clubs, Fundraisers, etc. Please contact our Special Sales Department.

To see Bragg Books and Products on-line, visit our Website at: www.bragg.com

 This book is printed on recycled, acid-free paper, which saves thousands of trees.

- REVISED AND EXPANDED -

Fifteenth Edition MMXI
ISBN: 978-0-87790-093-1

Library of Congress Cataloging-in-Publication Data on file with publisher

Published in the United States
HEALTH SCIENCE, Box 7, Santa Barbara, California 93102 USA

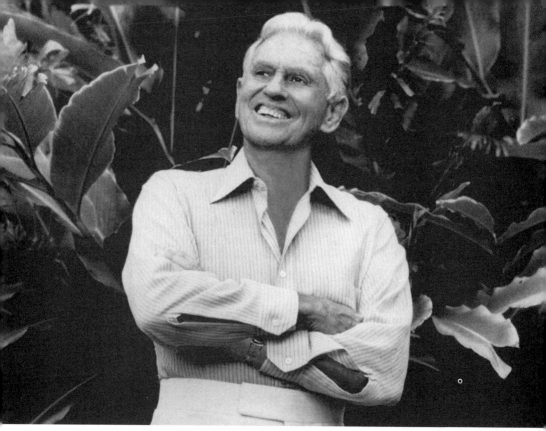

PAUL C. BRAGG, N.D., Ph.D.
World's Leading Healthy Lifestyle Authority

Paul C. Bragg's daughter Patricia and their wonderful, healthy members of the Bragg *Longer Life, Health and Happiness Club* exercise daily on the beautiful Fort DeRussy lawn, at famous Waikiki Beach in Honolulu, Hawaii. View club exercising *www.bragghawaiiexercise.com*. Membership is free and open to everyone to attend – Monday through Saturday, 9 to 10:30 am – for Bragg Super Power Breathing and Health and Fitness Exercises. On Saturday there are often health lectures on how to live a long, healthy life! The group averages 50 to 75 per day, depending on the season. From December to March it can go up to 125. Its dedicated leaders have been carrying on the class for over 40 years. Thousands have visited the club from around the world and have carried the Bragg Health and Fitness Crusade to friends and relatives back home. When you visit Honolulu, Hawaii, Patricia invites you and your friends to join her and the club for wholesome, healthy fellowship. She also recommends visiting the outer Islands (Kauai, Hawaii, Maui, Molokai) for a fulfilling, healthy vacation.

To maintain good health, normal weight and increase the good life of radiant health, joy and happiness, the body must be exercised properly (stretching, walking, jogging, running, biking, swimming, deep breathing, good posture, etc.) and nourished wisely with healthy foods. – Paul C. Bragg

iii

WE NEED YOUR SUPPORT!

With Your Support The Bragg Health Crusades Can Continue to Spread Paul C. Bragg's Teachings

For over 80 years we have been sharing Paul C. Bragg's teachings on healthy living worldwide! Millions are following the Bragg Healthy Lifestyle principles and their lives have been changed forever! Everyday people send us letters, e-mails and call, saying – *"Paul Bragg saved my life!"*

Former U.S. Surgeon General, Dr. C. Everett Koop said Paul Bragg did more for the Health of America than any one person he knew of.

OUR MISSION: To spread health worldwide and inspire youth and people of all ages to achieve optimal health – physically, mentally and spiritually and live long, productive, caring, happy lives.

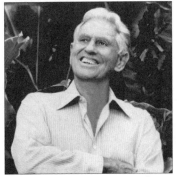

Paul C. Bragg, N.D., Ph.D.
Originator of Health Stores
Life Extension Specialist
Health Crusader to the World

If your life has been touched and helped by Bragg health teachings, please help us carry on the Bragg Legacy in this 21st Century and beyond. Your tax deductible donation to the *Bragg Health Institute* will support our mission to continue the Bragg Message of Health worldwide and inspire future generations.

The non-profit and philanthropic work of the *Bragg Health Institute* funds The *Bragg Health Crusades*, community health, health education lectures, health seminars, and publications on healthy living. The Institute conducts health outreach to youth in schools, also organic gardening teaching programs, and helps sponsor health science research and provides scholarships to worthy students pursuing the natural health science professions.

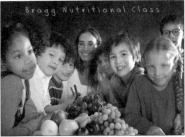

Bragg Outreach to Schools

Please join us in sharing The Bragg Health Legacy!

(Please see next page for more information)

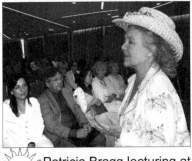

iv Patricia Bragg lecturing at Bragg Health Seminars

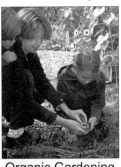

Organic Gardening Teaching Programs

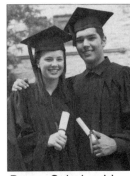

Bragg Scholarships

HEALTH DREAM WITH NEW HEALTH VISION

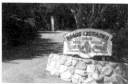
Health Institute Entrance

The Bragg Health Institute is located on a beautiful 120 acre Campus and Organic Farm on the Coast of Santa Barbara, California. Patricia Bragg and the Directors of Bragg Health Institute have designated this as the future site of the greatest living tribute to the life of Paul C. Bragg. The new Bragg Health Institute will become a world center for organic and healthy lifestyle education and research. (See our *Mission, Purpose and Vision for the Future* video on *bragghealthinstitute.org*)

You can also be part of Paul Bragg's lasting legacy by having your name inscribed upon one of the educational nature walks or inspirational walls of the Bragg Health Institute Campus and Organic Farm. Or you may want to have your name inscribed in the Grand Entrance or a room in the Bragg Memorial Library or Health Education Center or you can sponsor the Health Teaching DVDs to schools. Your name can be part of your own legacy, as you will be recognized for generations to come as a great Health Crusader because of your financial support of these wonderful health projects. When thousands of visitors see your name each year, they will know that you helped make a difference in the world.

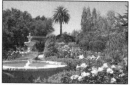
Visitor's Circle & Fountain

Some Special Health Projects You Can Partner with us:

- ❏ Healthy Lifestyle DVD's to Schools
- ❏ Scholarships for Future Health Doctors
- ❏ Teaching Medicinal Herb Gardens
- ❏ Paul Bragg Library & Rose Gardens
- ❏ Special Health Events & Programs
- ❏ Organic Teaching Gardens
- ❏ Health Teaching Kitchen
- ❏ Health Eco Education Center
- ❏ Bragg Nature & Farm Walks
- ❏ Bragg Health Museum

— — — — — — — — — — *COPY AND MAIL* — — — — — — — — — — — —

YES! I would like to help support Bragg Health Crusades by making a contribution to the Bragg Health Institute, a 501(c)(3) non-profit foundation, tax ID# 27-0983248 Your contributions are tax deductible.

❏ Enclosed is my tax-deductible gift of $_____ ○ Check ○ VISA ○ MC ○ Discover
   ○ $25 ○ $50 ○ $100 ○ $250 ○ $500 ○ $1,000 ○ $2,500 ○ $_____
❏ Please send me info on where my name can be permanently inscribed at Bragg Center.

My gift is in honor/memory of _____

Please send notice of this gift to (name & address):_____

_____

Credit Card Number:_____

Signature:_____

Card Expires: _____ / _____
month / year

Your Name   PLEASE PRINT

Address   Apt. No.

City   State   Zip

(____) _____
Phone   e-mail

If giving by check, please make check payable to: ***Bragg Health Institute***
Mail To: Box 7, Santa Barbara, CA 93102 USA • (805) 968-1020

For more info check out our web: www.bragghealthinstitute.org   V
Spreading health worldwide since 1912

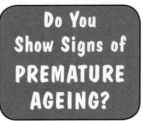

Do You Show Signs of PREMATURE AGEING?

Is everything you do a big effort?

•

Have you started to lose your skin tone? Your muscle tone? Your energy? Your hair?

•

Do small things irritate you? Are you forgetful? Confused?

•

Is your elimination sluggish?

•

Do you have allergies? Joint pains?

•

Do your feet hurt?

•

Do you have aches and pains?

•

Do you get out of breath when you run or climb stairs?

•

How limber is your back and body?

•

How well do you adjust to cold and heat?

•

Ask yourself these important questions: Am I healthy and happy? Do I seem to be slipping and not quite like myself anymore? If the answer to these questions are "Yes,"

START TODAY
Living The
Bragg Healthy
Lifestyle!

LOSS OF TEETH

HAIR OF • THINNING

FADING OF SIGHT

SALIVARY GLANDS SHRINK

LOSS OF HEARING

HIGH BLOOD PRESSURE

STIFFENING OF JOINTS

vi

He who understands and follows Mother Nature walks with God.

Build Powerful NERVE FORCE

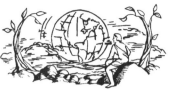

To preserve health is a moral and religious duty, for health is the basis for all social virtues. We can no longer be as useful when not well. – Dr. Samuel Johnson, Father of Dictionaries

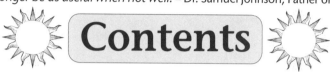

Contents

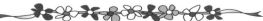

Open my eyes to see clearly the wonders of thy teachings. – Psalms 119:18

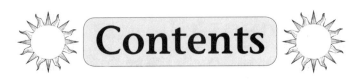

Contents

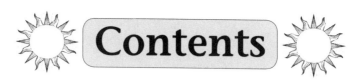

Contents

Chapter 4: Spiritual Health Promotes Physical Health. . 49

True wisdom consists in not departing from nature, but molding our conduct according to her wise laws. – Seneca

---

Throughout my life with my strong Nerve Force, I have received strength, enthusiasm and purpose of mind, body and soul.
– Paul C. Bragg, N.D., Ph.D., from *Awaken Health and Happiness*, 1937

Doubt destroys. Faith builds. – Robert Collier

When you sell a man a book you don't just sell him paper, ink and glue, you sell him a whole new life! There's heaven and earth in a real book. The real purpose of books is to trap the mind into its own thinking. – Christopher Morley

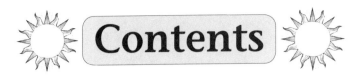

Contents

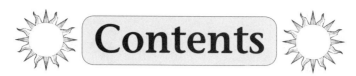

Contents

Chapter 6: Natural Healthy Food (continued)

You are what you eat, drink, breathe, think, say and do.
– Patricia Bragg, N.D., Ph.D., Pioneer Health Crusader

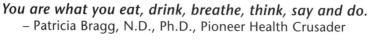

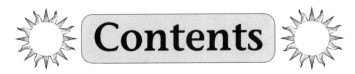

Contents

Breathing deeply, fully and completely energizes the body, calms the nerves, fills you with peace and helps keep you youthful. – Paul C. Bragg

It's never too late to be what you might have been. – George Elliot

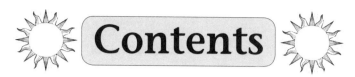

Contents

*Bragg Health Books are silent health teachers and your friends –
never tiring, ready night or day to help guide you to super health!*

Our habits, good or bad, are something we can control. – Dr. E. J. Stieglitz

*A horse that resists the reins, a car without brakes and a
person with no self-control, are all equally headed for disaster.*

The heart that loves is always young. – Greek proverb

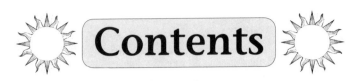

Contents

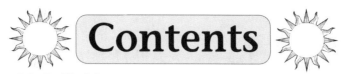

Contents

TEN HEALTH COMMANDMENTS

Thou shall respect and protect thy body as the highest manifestation of thy life.
Thou shall abstain from unnatural, devitalized foods and stimulating beverages.
Thou shall nourish thy body with only natural unprocessed, live foods, that . . .
Thou shall extend thy years in health for loving, sharing and charitable service.
Thou shall regenerate thy body by the right balance of activity and rest.
Thou shall purify thy cells, tissue and blood with healthy foods, and
    with clean air, gentle sunshine and pure water.
Thou shall abstain from all food when out of sorts in mind or body.
Thou shall keep thoughts, words and emotions pure, calm, loving and uplifting.
Thou shall increase thy knowledge of Mother Nature's Laws, follow them,
    and enjoy the fruits of thy life's labor.
Thou shall lift up thyself, friends and family by loyal dedicated obedience
    to Mother Nature's and God's Healthy, Natural Wise Laws of Living.

Why My Father & I Wrote This Book

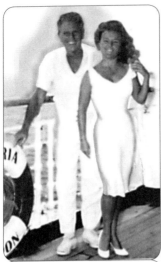

World Health Crusaders Paul C. Bragg and daughter, Patricia

Let us share with you our experiences with Powerful Nerve Force versus Nervous Fatigue. My father knows what it is to be so exhausted that every cell of your body seems to cry out with extreme weakness! He was once so ill and weak that he couldn't raise his head from a pillow. That changed because he changed his lifestyle.

Dad learned how to rebuild his Powerful Nerve Force the Natural Way and lived to be a great, great, grandfather with a vast storehouse of energy. We enjoy our ageless, tireless bodies and enjoy our busy lives and are getting more accomplished than ever before – yet we still have time to indulge in our many athletic hobbies. We've hiked the highest mountains in the world and can still play a fast game of tennis with people young enough to be our great grandchildren! We still swim and lift weights 3 times a week. We can ride our bikes or jog for miles at a time, then write books and at times travel off on the Bragg Health Crusades around the world.

This book outlines our Bragg Building Powerful Nerve Force Program. It can change your entire life! You will learn how to master your life with new zest for living and how to change nervous exhaustion into inexhaustible energy! You can build a new life for yourself if you follow our program faithfully . . . because your life and energy flows through your nerves! We can help, but it's your life and it's up to you!

xvi

Bragg Healthy Lifestyle Plan

- *Read, plan, plot, and follow through for supreme health and longevity.*
- *Underline, highlight or dog-ear pages as you read important passages.*
- *Organizing your lifestyle helps you identify what's important in your life.*
- *Be faithful to your health goals everyday for a healthy, long, happy life.*
- *Where space allows we have included "words of wisdom" from great minds to motivate and inspire you. Please share your favorite sayings with us.*
- *Write us about your successes following The Bragg Healthy Lifestyle.*

Chapter 1

What is Nerve Force?

Your Body's Command Center

It is the health and vitality of the millions of nerve cells that make up your vast nervous system. You need a powerful Nerve Force – stored in the numerous and varied nerve cells composing the nervous system – to attain and maintain the ideal balance for perfect super health. The nervous system consists of two sections controlled by a centralized command center – the brain:

1. THE EXTERNAL NERVOUS SYSTEM

Controls the skin surface and external muscles of the body. It transmits it to the brain's command center that governs movements of the arms, legs, head and other external muscles, as well as the skin's sensitivity to heat, cold and injury.

2. THE INTERNAL NERVOUS SYSTEM
Known as the Autonomic System – it has two subsystems, the sympathetic and the parasympathetic. These govern the internal functions of the body (i.e., the vital organs).

3. THE BRAIN
Acts as clearing house for the entire organism – the "control room" in which the mind "programs" the whole body's "computer system". It is interesting to note that according to scientists the human brain has a storage capacity of about 1,000 years.

It's suppose to be a professional secret, but I'll tell you anyway. We doctors do nothing. We only help and encourage the doctor within. – Albert Schweitzer

There is no wealth greater than the health of the body. – The Bible

Shocking Facts: *American healthcare costs soared to $600 billion back in 1991 and this is expected to go to $2.45 trillion by 2013. This is all the more reason each American should lead a Healthy Lifestyle to save our economy from this huge medical expense, not to mention the premature death and suffering (physical, mental, emotional and financial burdens).*

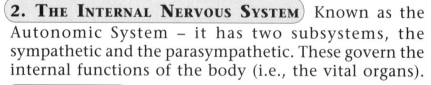

The Three Forms of Nerve Force

There are three forms of Nerve Force by which the human "network", your nervous system operates:

1. MUSCULAR NERVE FORCE: This is the Nerve Force that produces our muscular action. A high degree of this force is found in those insects and smaller animals which have tremendous muscular power in proportion to their size. An elephant could jump over mountains and push down the highest skyscraper if it possessed the same degree of Muscular Nerve Force as a flea, ant or small bug!

2. ORGANIC NERVE FORCE: The activity of our vital organs depends upon this form of Nerve Force. A high level of this Nerve Force produces robust health and the ability to resist disease. This leads to a long, peaceful, healthy life.

3. MENTAL NERVE FORCE: Essentially a mental quality, a powerful Mental Nerve Force that produces a keen intellect, good memory, mental endurance and a generally high psychic power. High Mental Nerve Force denotes a well-balanced, healthy person that has good control of their emotions. Stresses, strains and tensions do not plague them since they are the master of their own destiny. Their Mental Nerve Force is so high that they are impervious to petty nagging and other minor irritations which people of lower Mental Nerve Force try to impose upon them.

No one can drag you down from your high pedestal of bliss-consciousness when your Mental Nerve Force is high! You are never out of mental equilibrium. You are a natural human being who enjoys a constant mental state of bliss. You have mental poise. You live by knowledge and wisdom. You know true contentment and peace of mind. Relish it and treasure it!!!

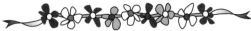

Ginkgo Biloba, the herb that improves blood flow through the brain and aids in mental acuity and stroke recovery, also appears to help normalize neuro-transmitter levels, and can help treat depression. In one European study, 80 mg. of ginkgo extract was given three times a day to a test group of 40 elderly individuals. After a few months, their depression lifted and their mental faculties improved significantly. However, if you use ginkgo, do not exceed 240 mg. per day, or you may develop some restlessness and irritability.

First we shape our environment and thereafter it shapes us. – Winston Churchill

Equilibrium of the Nervous System

In 1588, famous poet William Byrd expressed it so beautifully in his *Psalms and Sonnets:*

> *My mind to me is a kingdom;*
> *Such perfect joy therein I find,*
> *That it exceeds all other bliss*
> *That God and Nature hath designed.*

In everything, God and Mother Nature strive for perfect balance or equilibrium. When humans interfere with the balance of Nature they are in for trouble.

There are three main factors which disturb the equilibrium of the Nervous System: Nerve Depletion, Nerve Depression and Nerve Tension. We will use non-technical terms while discussing these afflictions because we want even the untrained student to understand each aspect of the topic. For example, when we refer to the Nervous System, we're generally alluding to the Internal (inner) and External (outer) workings.

3

Nerves are Pathways that Carry Vital Info Between Your Muscles, Organs and Brain.

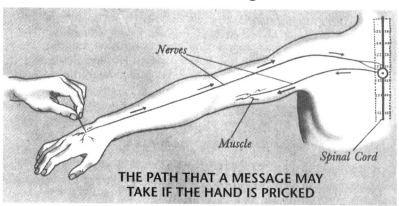

Nerves

Muscle

Spinal Cord

THE PATH THAT A MESSAGE MAY TAKE IF THE HAND IS PRICKED

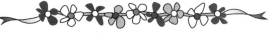

It is estimated that 23.6 million Americans are affected by diabetes. According to the American Diabetes Association, about 50% of those with diabetes have some form of nerve damage. The symptoms usually start with burning, throbbing, numbness or tingling in hands, legs or feet. These warnings are potentially dangerous and serious nerve damage can occur over several years. Oftentimes, pain medicines such as aspirin may not work with diabetic nerve pain. It's important to contact your health professional at the first signs of any symptoms.

Take Time for 12 Things

1. Take time to **Work** –
   it is the price of success.
2. Take time to **Think** –
   it is the source of power.
3. Take time to **Play** –
   it is the secret of youth.
4. Take time to **Read** –
   it is the foundation of knowledge.
5. Take time to **Worship** –
   it is the highway of reverence and
   washes the dust of earth from our eyes.
6. Take time to **Help and Enjoy Friends** –
   it is the source of happiness.
7. Take time to **Love and Share** –
   it is the one sacrament of life.
8. Take time to **Dream** –
   it hitches the soul to the stars.
9. Take time to **Laugh** –
   it is the laughing that helps life's loads.
10. Take time for **Beauty** –
    it is everywhere in nature.
11. Take time for **Health** –
    it is the true wealth and treasure of life.
12. Take time to **Plan** –
    it is the secret of being able to have time
    for the first 11 things.

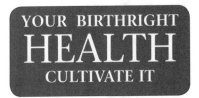

YOUR BIRTHRIGHT
HEALTH
CULTIVATE IT

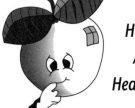

*Have an
Apple
Healthy Life!*

*Teach me Thy way O Lord, and
lead me in a simple plain path.* – Psalms 27:11

Chapter 2

Build Powerful Nerve Force

Nerve Force Is Your Vital Key to Life

My father and I love being health crusaders and make no attempt to produce literary classics when writing the Bragg Healthy Lifestyle books. We write in simple, easy-to-understand language and present health facts and wisdom that can be deeply imprinted upon the reader's mind to inspire them to live a healthy life. Our health message is of such vital importance that it should be brought to the attention of every man, woman and youth around the world.

We are living in the age of nerve stress. The terrific strain of the present-day "mile-a-minute rat race" is slowly but surely undermining the very foundations of our existence. Unless we take determined steps now to counter-act this threat, in a few decades we may find ourselves in a world populated with nervous wrecks! We are especially concerned for the American people. Throughout the world sufferers from nervous disorders abound, but it is American men, women and children who strain their nerves the most.

Our deep interest is in sharing this message of how to have healthy nerves, since each of us is governed by our Nerve Force. I am also interested in this subject because my father was born with highly sensitive nerves. I too have always had high energy, along with sensitive, active nerves. As a young man it became imperative for my father to learn to control his Nerve Force so he could reach his lifetime goal – being a health crusader!

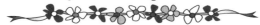

There is just one life for each of us: our own. – Euripides

You are what you eat, drink, breathe, think, say and do. – Patricia Bragg

---

Good health and good sense are two of life's greatest blessings.
– Publilius Syrus, 42BC

Remember, you are punished by your bad habits of living. – Paul C. Bragg

Paul Bragg Pioneered New Way to Health

After he had defeated tuberculosis at 18, Dad became intensely interested in healthy lifestyles and fitness and resolved to achieve the highest physical perfection allowed by Mother Nature. The developmental process of his study and practice of Health Culture began with physical exercise and athletics because he believed – as many do today – that muscular strength means health. As the fallacy of this dangerous theory became clear to him, he began to concentrate on scientific nutrition, deep breathing and systematic body-building to repair and renew his physique. He remained always on the alert to find the weakest cog in his body's machinery.

He found the most vulnerable factor in health to be the nerves, the body's governing force. That is where the body is weakest and most sensitive to abuse. We must begin to build up our Vital Nerve Force in the nerves! This statement is not based upon mere theory. Dad personally supervised Physical and Nutritional Programs for thousands yearly, also teaching thousands of students who attended our Bragg Health Crusades worldwide. The truths of my father's early teachings are now becoming accepted and honored by the top universities and health professionals worldwide.

The Secret of Nerve Force

Nerve Force is the source of all life! Life itself flows through your nerves – never forget that! When fully supplied with Nerve Force, we are enthusiastic, happy, fit and ambitious. We overcome difficulties and are ready to accept the challenges that life offers. Problems of all kinds become manageable when we are confident that we have Vital Nerve Force to cope with them.

People with powerful Nerve Force cannot be beaten. They rise up again for a new start, no matter how often they might fail. In the end, they win! Thus, 95% of humanity is dominated by the other 5%. It's Nerve Force that does the leading and makes the difference!

When health is absent, wisdom cannot reveal itself, strength cannot be exerted, wealth is useless and reason is powerless. – Herophiles, 300 B.C.

Nerve Force Is the Key to Vital Living

Your health, strength, vitality and endurance are directly measured by the degree of your Nerve Force. It gives you the reserve power that makes life successful and fascinating. The world is full of people with the brains and ability to rise to the top, but who lack the necessary Nerve Force to push them forward. A person's beauty, charm and vivacity are directly related to the Nerve Force that makes them sparkle with radiant health.

Your body is a complicated machine; Nerve Force and physical health are interdependent. Nerve Force is the driving power – but its generation, in turn, depends upon the harmonious activities of the vital organs. Your body is nourished throughout its every part by a vast circulatory system that carries oxygenated blood from your heart and lungs. If an organ is not functioning properly, your blood will not contain the elements necessary to create the right sort of Nerve Force. Your stomach must digest efficiently. The digestion assimilating process must be dependable. The eliminating organs – the bowels, lungs, kidneys and skin – must have tremendous Nerve Force to work efficiently. The spleen, liver and all the vital organs of the complex blood-making laboratory must all work harmoniously.

7

> If you arise every morning feeling dull and fatigued, if you are without ambition or goals, if you feel old, worn and dragged-out, or if the future looks hopeless and you feel defeated and helpless, then there's something wrong with your nervous system! Your Nerve Force is depleted and must be renewed! Good News: You don't have to feel this way! Read on - learn how to improve!

There is one thing you can do – start rebuilding your vital Nerve Force today! The body is a miraculous self-cleansing and self-healing organism when you give it and Mother Nature a chance. Unfortunately, most people, especially Americans today, are depleting their Nerve Force and are whipping their nerves in a desperate effort to compensate. This only makes everything worse.

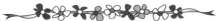

Over a 70 year lifespan, your busy stomach processes about 40 tons of food.

Perfect health is above gold; a healthy body before riches. – Solomon

"Bad Nerves" Are Dangerous and Are Destroying American Youth and Adults

"Bad Nerves . . ." We hear about them constantly and everywhere! The physician tells a patient, "It's your nerves." Sensitive and highly-strung people complain about their "nerves." Day after day you hear of housewives, blue-collar workers, business and professional people having a "nervous breakdown". You even hear parents say of their child, "He's so nervous, he won't listen to me and I can't discipline him!"

Teenagers are one of the most nervous groups of our entire population. Young peoples' nerves are so jangled that they require the pounding beat of rap or heavy metal music to stimulate them. Some must have it on constantly that they carry MP3 players with earbuds around with them to beat their exhausted nerves. They surf the web and watch violent movies, TV shows and videos. Millions are becoming heavy alcohol and drug users.

You see evidence of "Nerves" everywhere – on the street, on buses, in the movies, in schools and colleges, and especially in your home, with your own family. In some households the television is on continually from dawn to midnight. Unfortunately, people seem to crave TV now. Most people's nerves are so worn out that they can only be stimulated by the sight and the sound of violence, crime and murder. Movies, the TV shows and videos are the number one school for promoting crime, corrupted living, drugs, premarital sex, early pregnancy and alcohol and drug abuse. TV shows with violent and sexual content have almost replaced the cultural and wholesome programs offered on TV. (Please complain – email, call.)

America is a nation of nervous people, a fact known the world over and openly admitted by our own nerve specialists. Our national intensity is directly related to our "mile-a-minute" lifestyle that causes nerve burnout! It's making us the most progressive nation on earth . . . but it's also destroying our health! Our crowded mental institutions prove this. Half of the hospital beds of the country are occupied by people with nervous disorders!

Who is strong? He that can conquer his bad habits. – Benjamin Franklin

There Is No Mental Health Without Powerful Healthy Nerve Force

The best authorities on mental health say that if mental illness continues to increase at the present rate, in less than a hundred years there will be no one to take care of the mentally ill because everybody will be the victim of some mental disorder! Sounds frightening, doesn't it? Medical records prove it. There are not enough psychiatrists and psychologists to handle the mentally ill today. America is in a sad and deplorable situation!

Millions of people have subnormal Nerve Force and as a consequence suffer from endless organic and physical troubles which make their lives miserable. When people don't have the Nerve Force or basic vitality to meet the pressure which life puts upon them, what happens? Let's take a look. The first thing most people do is to take one of the milder stimulants – such as tobacco, coffee, tea, candy or cola drinks – to combat their stress. The deeper their Nerve Force reserves drop, the more often they seek out the stronger stimulants – alcohol and harder drugs. It is not long before far too many of them become addicted to some dangerous and powerful drug.

There are many people who consider themselves normal, yet they cannot go through an ordinary day without the use of some kind of pill. At night their nerves are so exhausted that they can't get rest without a sleeping pill! Just watch your TV and note how many pain, sleeping and tranquilizers pills are advertised!

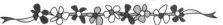

Even in Australia, total cost of workers compensation claims for stress-related conditions is over $200 million every year! – betterhealth.vic.gov.au

---

*Americans fill more than 3.4 billion prescriptions a year.
– Center for Disease Control & Prevention*

---

*Yesterday is the past. Tomorrow's the future. But today is a gift . . .
That is why it is called the present.*

---

*Life is a gift – open it. A joy – share it. A game – play it.
An experience – live it. A dream – make it come true!*

Dear friend, I wish above all things that thou may prosper and be in health, even as the soul prospers. – 3 John 2

Why Are There Alcohol & Drug Problems?

Our daily newspapers are filled with accounts of young men and women of high school and college age abusing themselves with alcohol, cocaine, etc. Medical authorities say that cocaine, crack and ecstasy are brain, body and health destroying drugs! Yet millions of nerve–depleted young Americans are using these drugs regularly! The same is true of marijuana, called "pot". Thousands of pounds are consumed by Americans daily. In fact, this "pot" habit is becoming so widespread that groups are promoting and legalizing this powerful nerve-destroying drug. Anything that gives the depleted nerves a *kick* is used by desperate *junkies*. Some Americans even sniff gasoline or glue and lapse into a stupor. We all know the tragic life these legal drugs – tobacco and alcohol cause millions of Americans. Some become addicted at an early age. There's 55 million smokers and over 76 million people who have a family member who is or was an alcoholic!

Visit webs: *www.lungusa.org* • *www.dfaf.org*
www.alcoholics-anonymous.org • *www.drugfree.org*

10

What is Meant by "Nerves"?

The popular expression "nerves" can actually mean Nerve Exhaustion or lack of Nerve Force. To ask, "What is Nerve Force?" one might as well ask, "What is Electricity?" Both are just as intangible. We know that Nerve Force is the Vital Force of Life, a mysterious energy that flows from the nervous system to give life and energy to every vital organ. Sever the nerve which leads to any organ and the organ will cease functioning.

The wonderful structure we term the Nervous System consists of millions of cells which act as reservoirs of Nerve Force. The amount of stored energy represents our Nerve Capital. Every organ works incessantly to keep the supply of Nerve Force in these cells at a high level. Life itself depends more upon Nerve Force than upon the food we eat or even the air we breathe. Without the activating Nerve Force we could neither breathe nor eat!

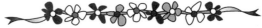

Alcohol abuse and Alcoholism are tragically the third leading cause of preventable deaths in the United States.

Depleting Our Reservoir of Nerve Force

There are numerous ways we unduly tax our nerves: poor nutrition, lack of oxygen or regular sleep, stress, overwork, anger, worry, jealousy, hate, envy, greed, self-pity, guilt and grief. If we subject our muscular system to excessive strain and consume more Nerve Force than the body can produce, the natural result is Nerve Bankruptcy: complete Nerve Exhaustion and maybe even a nervous breakdown! There is but one malady more terrible than Nervous Exhaustion – its kin, insanity! Those who have endured this know the terrible suffering involved. Nervous Exhaustion can put a cloud of misery over your life.

The Danger Signals of Low Nerve Force

When the Nerve Force is low, you can go through life burdened with fear and never recognize its presence. Only a courageous self-analysis will disclose the presence of this universal enemy. When you begin such an analysis, search deeply into your character and be brutally honest with yourself! As you will note, the symptoms of fear and low Nerve Force themselves will work against such honesty. You must collect and redirect your remaining Nerve Force to head-off these danger signals! It's your first step onto the Road of High Health. *Check For:*

1. INDIFFERENCE: Do you tend to easily accept, without protest, whatever life offers you? Do you lack initiative, imagination, enthusiasm and self-control? Low Nerve Force drains away your ambition, while it's making you mentally and physically lazy, willing to tolerate poverty or a lower standard of living. It also makes you unable to get out of a demeaning situation.

2. INDECISION: Are you inclined to let others do your thinking for you? Would you rather be led than make decisions for yourself? A person with low Nerve Force is easily brainwashed because others can control their mind. They can actually become a human robot who does not question anything, even their own actions!

"Why not look for the best – the best in others, the best in ourselves, the best in all life situations? He who looks for the best knows the worst is there, but refuses to be discouraged by it. Life will soon become more pleasant for you and everyone around you." – Rev Paul S. Osumi, Hawaii

3. DOUBT: Do you secretly doubt your ability to do things and as a consequence, also doubt the sincerity of those who want to help you? Low Nerve Force is often characterized by excuses designed to cover up, explain away or apologize for personal failures. It is sometimes expressed in the form of criticism or envy of those who have sparkling health or those who have found success in life.

4. WORRY: Are you a chronic worrier? This is a major danger signal of low Nerve Force and can easily lead to a nervous breakdown! Worriers are miserable people, living in a haze of fears. Worrying saps the life out of a person and ages them prematurely. It is an absolute and scientific fact that you can worry yourself into the hospital and an early grave!

If your Nerve Force is low to the point of chronic worry, you will probably say, "If you had my problems, you would worry, too!" That is not necessarily true. Everyone encounters problems as life goes on – often bigger ones than you have encountered. But a person who has powerful Nerve Force does not worry about a problem. They face it objectively and in a calm, logical, practical way they find a solution! Often, after carefully examining a problem and if they are unable to find a solution, they will turn it over to a Higher Power and pray for the answer. We have seen miracles with prayer!

Worrying about a problem will not solve it! It only destroys your health and ages you prematurely. Worry is a killer! Build a strong Nerve Force and solutions come.

5. BEING OVERLY CAUTIOUS: Do you wait for "the right time" to begin putting ideas and plans into action – until waiting becomes a permanent habit? When Nerve Force is low, pessimism is high. One habitually looks for the negative side of every situation – thinking and talking of possible failure instead of concentrating upon the means of success. This leads to knowing all the roads to disaster but never searching for ways and means to avoid failure. Constant procrastination and uncertainty often leads to tension, poor circulation, indigestion, constipation, nervousness, bad breath and a terrible disposition.

No man can violate Nature's Laws and escape her penalties! – Julian Johnson

A Healthy Lifestyle is The Wisest and Best Remedy for Nervous Disorders

Let it be definitely understood that we can't offer any cures for nervous conditions. We do not prescribe, diagnose or treat disease in any way. That is strictly for the doctors. We are teachers instructing people in a Program of Natural Living that will keep their entire body in good physical condition. This program – The Bragg Healthy Lifestyle – includes correct daily habits of eating, exercising, sleeping, breathing, fasting, relaxing, bathing, posture, and even a technique of meditation for developing powerful control over the mind and body. Everyone who wishes to be free from chronic fatigue and build powerful Nerve Force must have full control of both their mind and body.

Live as Mother Nature Intended You to Live!

One of the dominant themes of this book is a gradual return to a more natural way of living. In your thinking, eating and all of your daily habits, you must strive for **13** simplicity of life. Try to reach a nearness to Mother Nature and make yourself at home with her. When you feel that the same pure forces which express themselves in a beautiful pine tree are manifesting themselves in you, then you have made a big stride toward the ideal life.

Begin to live as Mother Nature and God want you to live. Seek and feel their love and know that you can be part of their healthy world-wide family. In your daily meditations repeat over and over again, "I am becoming the perfect child of God and Mother Nature!" You become one with Mother Nature when you live the natural Bragg Healthy Lifestyle. As you become a part of Mother Nature in body, mind, and spirit, you will then be able to attain the highest possible Nerve Force!

Strong Hearts, Nerves and Minds

New Study (www.time.com) shows people with weak pumping hearts had decreased brain volume – a sign of brain ageing. Even small reductions in blood flow to the brain may speed ageing and has potential to compromise cognitive function. Start living Bragg Healthy Lifestyle and read Bragg Heart Book.

Happiness and Love are Simplicity

Happiness and Love are what we all seek, and when found, life can be heaven on earth! Let's be like children – pleased with simple things! The more we complicate our lives, the more we drain our Nerve Force. With wholesome health and serenity of mind, let us live our lives in tranquility and contentment! Let us find the pure joy of living! Let us love Mother Nature as she reveals herself to us in all her simplicity and beauty! If we live a useful, humble, sane life according to her righteous laws – cultivating happiness and sharing it with those near and dear to us – we will do more than well! The best religion of all is found in kindness, understanding, giving and sharing. The real measure of our sunshine is in the brightness we can kindle in the eyes of others.

Love and Survival

Famous Dr. Dean Ornish *(ornish.com)*, states how you feel emotionally can affect your health physically . . .

14

> *In my work with cardiac patients over the last 30 years, I am convinced that love and intimacy are at the root of health and illness; there is such a thing as the healing power of love!*

UC Berkeley Scientists studied patients who were undergoing coronary angiography. Those who felt the most loved and supported by family and friends, had substantially less blockage in the heart arteries. These findings are similar in Swedish research. More than 1,700 men and women between the ages of 29 and 74, were studied for 6 years. Those who were more isolated with low emotional support were four times more at risk of dying prematurely. Clearly, scientific studies have proven that the capacity to nurture and be nurtured – to have a loving heart is a vital link to a long and healthy life!

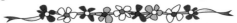

Many people treat their bodies as if they were rented from Hertz – something they are using just to get around in, but nothing they genuinely care about understanding. – Chungliang Al Huang

You cannot attain healthy relaxation in the true sense of the word when you use toxic stimulants and nerve destroying drugs. – Exercise for Health

If we will only let her, Mother Nature will comfort us and bring us joy. Let us try to understand her with the minds of servants . . . but enjoy her with the open and glad hearts of children. To have overall powerful Nerve Force we must learn the great Laws of Mother Nature and live by them. That is what this book is all about. Its purpose is to show you how to live by the Laws of Mother Nature and God and reap the rewards of Health and Happiness. The kingdom of heaven is within you! Make your heaven here and now!

By trusting in Mother Nature and obeying her laws, understanding your physical machinery and the way to care for it, you can build a powerful Nerve Force that can bring you unbelievable happiness! No matter how low you feel mentally, physically, spiritually and emotionally, know that the body is a self-cleansing, self-repairing, and self-healing instrument. Give your body a chance and its recuperating vital forces can make you a new healthy, happy, fulfilled person!

The Art of Long, Healthy, Happy Living

One of the best recipes for a long, healthy and happy life is just to keep on living by God's and Mother Nature's Laws. Consider each day as a little life in itself and make it as perfect and well-rounded as you possibly can.

What you sow in one period of your life, you reap in another. Live well today so you will have a better tomorrow! Try to be better physically and mentally on your next birthday than you are now. By living supremely for the moment you are investing in a superb life for your future. However, please be aware of yourself! The moment you relax your guard, the enemy is ready to rush in and smite your weak spot. A few may live long and happily without trying to live well and healthfully, but you will live longer, be healthier and happier if you make a conscious effort! Living for health, longevity and happiness is an art. If you deliberately strive to prolong your life in health and happiness, you may just do so!

In recent study researchers found obese people are more likely to have mental health problems. Poor physical health can lead to issues with low self-esteem and body image, which increases anxiety and depression.

Build Your Own Nerve Force

The reason we told you we offer no magic cures for people with nerve problems is because to build powerful Nerve Force you, and you alone, must do it! It is day to day living and thinking that is important. We will outline our entire Bragg Healthy Lifestyle for you in this book, but we cannot live it for you – nor can anyone else! No one can eat, exercise, fast, breathe or meditate for you. The more you put into this Nerve Force Program, the more good benefits you will reap from it!

Our Program is designed to not only give you powerful Nerve Force, it will also make you a more balanced person physically and mentally. The program is designed to lead you to "bliss consciousness", which simply means getting more out of your life – more peace, serenity and happiness. This is the true joy of living!

This Is Your Life To Love and Protect

You were put here to enjoy life! And though we firmly believe that the kingdom of heaven is within every person, we also believe that you must work to reach that heavenly state of joyful living! We must earn it! It is not handed out on a silver platter. Remember that what you give to life is what you get from life. The results you will get out of The Bragg Healthy Lifestyle will be in exact proportion to the effort you put into it.

Nerve Force is the most precious gift of God and Mother Nature. It means everything – your happiness, your health and your success in life. You must learn all there is to know about your nerves: how to protect, relax, calm and soothe your nerves. In this way, you can rebuild your precious Nerve Force, as you strive to keep yourself healthy, physically and mentally fit.

The *Archives of General Psychiatry* cites recent studies that show how stress markedly delays wound healing. One study assessed the relationship between the psychological stress and the secretion of pro-inflammatory cytokines – development of local immune responses that are central in the early stages of wound repair. Researchers induced skin blisters on the forearms of 36 women. Those with higher perceived stress scores had lower level of cytokines production, causing slow healing.

Worry and Stress Are Killers

Nerve and stress related diseases occur world-wide. In China, heart disease and stroke are projected to increase by 73% by the year 2030 or sooner! The country will lose $558 billion to these stress-related diseases, according to the World Health Organization. As in many parts of the world, decreased physical activity and unhealthy diets are leading to obesity, increased blood pressure and cholesterol and diabetes which leads ultimately to cardiac problems (see web: *www.bloomberg.com*).

Most humans are so full of worry that they believe they can never overcome their miseries. Each day the little bit of Nerve Force they have is dissipated by worrying about their difficulties. This is one sure way to arrive at a complete nervous breakdown. The surest way to become a nervous wreck is to worry. Worrying about a problem does not solve it – it only makes things worse. As we said before, you can literally "worry yourself to death". A Hollywood neighbor of ours almost did!

Suicide Rate Soaring Among All Ages!

This woman had multiple serious problems. She suffered with migraine headaches that almost drove her crazy. She was chronically constipated, tortured by insomnia and gas pains. Her husband was an alcoholic. Their two children were wild, uncontrollable teenagers who brought her and her husband nothing but grief. She was worried to the breaking point and had thoughts of committing suicide. Records show in America, thousands resort to suicide to escape from their worries, and suicide rates are soaring even among teenagers. The main causes are: the crime, killing and death that is promoted in movies, TV, the web, videos and rap music (parental controls on TV and computer important). Also the unhealthy, immoral lifestyles of youth are often due to a lack of parental and spiritual guidance that should and could provide a solid foundation for a well-balanced life!

Many people go through their life committing partial suicide.
They destroy their health, youth, talents, energies and creative qualities.
Indeed, to learn how to be good to oneself is often harder than
to learn how to be good to others. – Joshua Liebman, Ph.D.

The Bragg Healthy Lifestyle Prevents Suicide

Finally, this neighbor came to our home one evening and told us what she had in mind. Naturally we told her this was a terrible thing to do to herself. We knew she could overcome her problems if she would follow Mother Nature's Laws. We told her that no matter what her worries were, we believed that if she would build her Nerve Force she could find the answers to most of her problems. We also told her that she had attempted to break every law of health and natural hygiene. By breaking these laws she had only succeeded in destroying her own physical, emotional and mental health!

We finally told her that we had no magic cures to offer her. All we could do was give her our complete Nerve Force Program and Bragg Healthy Lifestyle, which both obey God's and Mother Nature's Eternal Laws!

The first thing about The Bragg Healthy Lifestyle we outlined for our neighbor was a fast of 3 days (page 116), allowing nothing but distilled water. We told her to leave home and go to some quiet spot in the country where she could enjoy absolute rest during this cleansing, recharge time.

18

From Nervous Breakdown To Health Buildup

She went to Lake Arrowhead, California and rented a cozy cabin among the big pines, and went on a complete three day distilled water fast. As she flushed the toxic poisons out of her body, she became calmer and was able to see her problems more objectively. This period of body purification made tremendous changes physically, spiritually, emotionally and mentally in her well-being. Her thinking was fresher, clearer, happier and healthier. She could take a overall bird's-eye view of her problems and start solving them, prayerfully one at a time.

The alcohol habit is the most harmful to the body and must be stopped! The Center for Disease Control & Prevention states excessive alcohol consumption is the 3rd largest cause of death after smoking and obesity. Alcohol fosters cancer in the body and even moderate drinking is risky to your health!!!

To preserve health is a moral and religious duty, for health is the strong basis for all social virtues. We can no longer be as useful when not well.
– Dr. Samuel Johnson, Father of Dictionaries, 1755

We outlined for our neighbor The Bragg Healthy Lifestyle eating program that eliminates all coffee, tea and unhealthy, devitalized foods. We put her on a healthy vegetarian diet for a full month. We told her to meditate and pray for 30 minutes in the morning and again at night. During these calm meditations she was to repeat the following affirmations, many times at first:

- *I have mind-heart-soul power to solve all my problems.*
- *My body is pure, clean and healthier from my detox fast.*
- *I'm now thinking constructively, not destructively!*

Instead of worrying about problems, she sought the answers in calm meditation. As she continued to rebuild her vitality, we introduced her to the complete Nerve Force Building Program detailed in this book. With a 24 hour fast (page 116) each week and The Bragg Healthy Lifestyle diet, her physical problems soon faded away. She began taking her husband to the *AA – Alcoholics Anonymous* meetings *(www.aa.org)* and this solved his drinking problem. This experience helped her as well. She realized the founders of AA had recognized the role of Nerve Force in helping to solve one of the major problems of our times – alcoholism! She also found it helped her, as it did other AA members at the opening of each meeting or during her own private meditations to recite and follow this wise world famous Sanskrit prayer:

Give me the Serenity to accept what cannot be changed; the Courage to change what can be changed; and the Wisdom to know the difference.

This woman also developed the Nerve Force necessary to cope with her two teenage children. She was now better equipped to communicate with them; something she had not been able to do for years. She found she could bridge the generation gap and find the essential common ground to meet and hold discussions with her children. Both of them made a big turn around, went on to college, got splendid grades and good jobs.

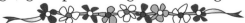

By changing personal behavior, we can reduce our risk of dying early by 70% to 80%. – John Graham, President, Professional Society for Risk Analysis

A well-spent day brings happy sleep. – Leonardo da Vinci

19

Keep Your Nerves Healthy and Strong

So someone who was ready to destroy herself got a new lease on life by turning to Natural Living and simply following the Laws of Mother Nature and God. We were only guides to help her to help herself! That is what we want to do for you, the reader of this book! We want to teach you how to build powerful Nerve Force by following the Eternal Laws of God and Mother Nature. Remember that life flows through your nerves. An alert and active nervous system is therefore the greatest gift of Mother Nature, for it is through the nerves that we experience the pleasures that make life wonderful and worth living. To be dull-nerved means to be mentally and physically dull – insensitive to the higher phases of life, incapable of deep emotions such as love, and lacking the spark-force of character and life.

It is true that highly sensitive and active nerves – when abused – are a menace to health. But don't consider it a misfortune if you are born with "high-energy" nerves. Although this means you must be wise in words and actions, for you could "explode" if you don't use caution. Before speaking put it to the test: Is it kind? Is it good? Is it necessary? This Program is designed to help you control your nerves and build a powerful Nerve Force – and use it wisely!

Two Sides of the Shield – Physical & Mental

The story is told of two knights who fought a duel to the death over the exact color of their King's shield which hung high above the center of his castle's great hall. One knight claimed that his sovereign's shield was red. The other asserted just as vehemently that it was green. After their tragic battle someone looked up at the shield – one side was green, the other side was red. Similarly there are two sides to the Shield of Health – the physical and the mental – both equally important!

It's sad to note for centuries the problem of health has been approached primarily on the physical level. Now we know we must do everything in our power not

Do what you can to improve, with what you have, where you are!
– Theodore Roosevelt, 26th American President, 1933–1945

only to keep ourselves physically fit, but also to keep ourselves mentally fit! You will accomplish the first goal by following our Nerve Force Program and The Bragg Healthy Lifestyle. You'll address the second by practicing your daily meditations and prayer, during which you must examine your body – inner and outer self – using reason, logic, intelligence to seek and find the answers to your long-term and daily problems.

A Strong Mind in a Strong Body

These two states – the physical and mental – are so closely interrelated that it is impossible to separate them. Physical health affects mental alertness and mental control imposes the necessary discipline to maintain physical health. For perfect health – including powerful Nerve Force – we must have a strong mind in a strong body. Flesh is dumb! Flesh does not operate through intelligence and reasoning, but through the five senses. Your body's first reaction in response to stimuli is to gratify the senses, such as satisfying hunger: for example, eating something that is pleasing to the taste, regardless of negative health benefits. A vicious circle can evolve into an unhealthy body and mind. The devitalized popular foods in our American diet fail to supply the proper nourishment! Flesh becomes weary, and Nerve Force becomes depleted on "foodless" fast junk foods.

Instead of seeking help from Mother Nature's healthy foods, human flesh seeks quick gratification from the temporary, but false sense of well-being provided by coffee, tea, sugar, colas, pills, alcohol or tobacco, etc. This gratification is temporary relief only! It causes further energy depletion, which can lead to stronger drug use that can create the "false illusions" of feeling good.

Now, your reason and intelligence will tell you that unhealthy living is slow bodily suicide! Since the brain is your body's "miracle captain" computer, reckless living causes mental deterioration! To build a strong body, the mind must be strong enough to assume control of the body, and establish and faithfully maintain The Bragg Healthy Lifestyle habits. A beneficial cycle will then ensue, for a healthy body is your best insurance for a healthy mind and powerful, healthy Nerve Force!

A strong mind will generate positive thoughts and help to keep the body on the High Road to Health. However, the mind can also produce negative thoughts and suggestions, so your mind must be strong enough to resist these impulses. A properly functioning body should have a mechanical precision that protects it from negative mental interference. Our first duty, therefore, must be to educate our bodies to follow The Bragg Healthy Lifestyle. As we improve the physical part of our human machinery, we will also improve our mental state. The brain demands five times as much blood as any other of our organs. Give it what it needs – healthy nutrition, exercise, deep breathing and do it with faithfulness – it will be grateful and perform better!

Make Your Body Worry Proof

The Greeks created this perfect phrase for this human interrelationship: **A strong mind in a strong body.** No one said it better. If you're mentally upset, you can walk miles – but if physically sick, then clear, constructive thinking is virtually impossible. By raising your physical health standards, your mental abilities will increase accordingly. Be on good terms with your body to enjoy your mind fully.

If our mental machinery is sluggish, we look to our physical machinery for explanations. What is the reason and the remedy for our halting thoughts and stumbling sentences? We usually find we need a break and some exercise. We refresh and recharge with a long, brisk walk, deeply breathing in the fresh air that cleans the cobwebs from our brains! When our mental creativity returns, then we return to our writing, the words flow effortlessly from our brains to the tips of our fingers – it's exciting. Dad and I love sharing our wisdom with you!

A merry heart is good medicine: but a broken spirit destroys health.
"A merry heart is healthful, but one that is broken in spirit and dejected will develop many bodily illnesses. Nothing ruins health faster than grief, anger, bad temper, jealousy, hatred, anxiety, worry and malice. We should cleanse and rid ourselves of all bad habits." – Proverbs 17:22

An Australian study found that female dementia rates could double in the next 20 years! Key factors are increased anxiety and depression, which are the biggest burdens on women's health. Nearly half the women in the study were found to be overweight, and to have high blood pressure.
Check website: www.perthnow.com.au

There Is No Reward For Worry

Most abnormal states of the mind can be traced to a malfunctioning nervous system, toxins in the blood or other physical causes. The famous Brain Research Institute, UCLA Medical School in Los Angeles is doing extensive research to determine as precisely as possible the physical causes of mental illnesses. Web: *bri.ucla.edu/*

We have always believed that abnormal mental states have physical explanations. Cheerfulness may be the result of sunshine communicating a sense of well-being to the cortical area of the brain. A tranquil scene will sometimes calm you by acting on your nervous system. A harmonious interior design may soothe the mind through the five senses.

Smiling is a great example of the close interaction between the mental and the physical states. We smile naturally when we are feeling happy. Have you ever tried making yourself smile when you are feeling blue? Try it! Physical acts of smiling *(takes 13 muscles)* and also laughing nearly always triggers mental reactions that makes you feel better! Don't forget it requires mental effort in the first place to make you "smile away your tears"!

Let's make a strong pledge to use the necessary mental discipline it takes to establish and maintain the physical discipline making the body "worry proof" (impervious to negative thoughts)! This will help to keep our minds healthy and free from worry. Educate the brawn and train the brain! You will then attain the healthier ideal balance for both – perfect physical and mental health.

Help with Panic Attacks

Panic attack episodes are intense fear or apprehension that are of sudden, yet brief duration. The most common symptoms may include trembling; chest pain; nausea and hyperventilation. Vitamin B deficiency and an unhealthy lifestyle may be major causes! Medical researchers at Mayo Clinic concluded 2 alternative therapies have the potential in the treatment of panic disorder: 1) Relaxation Training – such as yoga, prayer, meditation and deep breathing. 2) Inositol Supplement: influences the action of Serotonin, which helps reduce the frequency and severity of panic attacks.

Good Posture Promotes Healthier Nerves

Look at yourself in the mirror. Do your shoulders slump? Is your upper back round? Do you have a protruding potbelly? Are you a swayback? Can you see the reasons why your back has the right to ache? The bending, slumping, ligament-stretching and the force of gravity has taken its toll. If you are a backache sufferer due to weak muscles and bad posture, (see page 25) don't despair, you can restore back comfort with this simple posture exercise (see below), The Bragg Healthy Lifestyle and read *Bragg Back Fitness* Book (see pages 211-213).

It has often been said that backache is the penalty man must pay for the privilege of standing and walking upright on two feet, often wearing uncomfortable shoes. Every infant struggles to stand instinctively on his own two feet and walk. He need not be taught. He will attempt this bipedal gait even if left alone most of the time and never instructed. It is natural for a human being to stand and walk in this manner. This is interesting, because there are no animals which spend all of their standing and walking hours on two feet, not even gorillas or chimpanzees. These apes use their hands and arms to help them move about. The world's strongest gorilla would be unable to follow a busy person, walking erectly, for more than a short time. This is because human beings were created and are meant to walk erect and animals are not.

Bragg Posture Exercise Gives Instant Youthfulness

Stand (feet 8" apart) before a mirror and stretch up your spine. Tighten buttocks and suck in stomach muscles, lift up rib cage, put chest out, shoulders back, and chin up slightly. Line body up straight (nose plumbline straight to belly button), drop hands to sides and swing arms to normalize your posture. Do this posture exercise daily and miraculous changes will happen! You are retraining and strengthening your muscles to stand straight for health and youthfulness. Remember when you slump, you also cramp your precious machinery. This posture exercise (do 2-3 times daily) will retrain your frame to sit, stand and walk tall for health, fitness and longevity!

Positive affirmations create miracles. – Beatrex Quntanna

WHERE DO YOU STAND?

POSTURE CHART

	PERFECT	FAIR	POOR
HEAD			
SHOULDERS			
SPINE			
HIPS			
ANKLES			
NECK			
UPPER BACK			
TRUNK			
ABDOMEN			
LOWER BACK			

Your posture carries you through life from your head to your feet. This is your human vehicle and you are truly a miracle! Cherish, respect and always protect it by living The Bragg Healthy Lifestyle. – Patricia Bragg

Good posture helps prevent backaches and related problems.

Remember – Your posture can make or break your health!

Start Building Your Nerve Force Today!

1. **Put a stop to all undue nerve waste.** Use prayer and meditation to clear mind of worries, fears, negative thoughts and emotions that drain away nerve energy. Replace these with a clear statement of your goal. See image of yourself as you want to become and with the confidence that you will achieve your purpose. Maintain a positive attitude that will greatly assist you in building powerful Nerve Force. See pages 49-66.

2. **Get 8 hours of deep, restful sleep every night.** Lower your stress levels and when possible take power naps and short siesta after midday meal. See pages 67-80.

3. **Adopt a program of eating that will keep you internally clean and healthy.** Give up all devitalized foods, drinks and all artificial stimulants: tobacco, alcohol, cola drinks, coffee, tea, salt, refined sugars, etc., and eat a preponderance of organic fruits and vegetables – both raw and lightly cooked. Fast 24 hours weekly taking only distilled water and the vinegar drink (page 41). Take a 7 to 10 day fast yearly to help unburden your nerves of all toxic poisons, obstructions and build-ups of any kind. See 81-116.

4. **Have a daily exercise program.** Get out in fresh air and exercise to improve circulation and sleep better. Walk briskly, jog, jump rope, swim, dance, do tai chi, chi gong and play games. Keep your 640 body muscles active and healthy! Buy a pedometer – fun to monitor walks, runs, etc. See pages 117-128.

5. **Breathe deeply.** Get more life-giving oxygen deep down in the lower lungs. Oxygen is your greatest "Nerve Tonic." Nerve Force is built with oxygen. The raw fruits and vegetables in your diet are loaded with oxygen, and taking purifying fasts will increase your body's capacity for absorbing oxygen. Through deep breathing you cleanse your blood of poisonous carbon dioxide and fill it with oxygen, which is taken to every cell in your body. See pages 129-138.

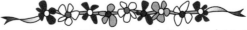

I am going to obey the Wise Laws of God and Mother Nature. I know I will find more health, peace of mind, joy and serenity.

6. **Bathe daily.** Drench your body with hot and cold water to increase your circulation, then enjoy healing rays of gentle sunlight. See pages 139-148.

7. **Keep your emotions under control.** Do not subject your nerves to stress that can be avoided. It is difficult enough to face and overcome the trials that you cannot avoid without going forth to seek other means of exhausting your nerves! See 149-158.

8. **Relax your nerves.** The natural rhythm of life is tension, then relaxation – like the beat of your heart. Strive to make your nervous system so powerful and healthy that your body will automatically shift from tension to relaxation. See pages 159-164.

9. **Enjoy life.** Don't forget to play and have fun as life goes on! That is one of the reasons you are here on earth – to enjoy it. Success and material possessions are all right in their place, but you must enjoy life each day to the fullest. Whistle, hum, sing, laugh and dance! Please keep away from dispensers of gloom. This old world has been a madhouse since **27** it first began. Do everything you can to make it a healthier, safer world and help improve yourself, family and friends and then others. See pages 165-168.

Morning Resolve To Start Your Day

I will this day live a simple, sincere and serene life; repelling promptly every thought of impurity, discontent, anxiety, discouragement and fear. I will cultivate health, cheerfulness, happiness, charity and the love of brotherhood; exercising economy in expenditure, generosity in giving, carefulness in conversation and diligence in appointed service. I pledge fidelity to every trust and a childlike faith in God. In particular, I will be faithful in those habits of prayer, study, work, nutrition, physical exercise, deep breathing and good posture. I shall fast for a 24 hour period each week, eat only healthy foods and get sufficient sleep each night. I will make every effort to improve myself physically, mentally, emotionally and spiritually every day.

Morning Prayer used by Paul C. Bragg and Patricia Bragg

YOUR STRESS SCALE TEST

Take This Quick Stress Quiz:

Indicate how strongly you agree with each of the following statements on a scale from 0 to 3:

0 = never 1 = sometimes 2 = often 3 = always

__ I have trouble relaxing.

__ I get frustrated when people are incompetent.

__ I feel tense and rushed.

__ I worry about work and other problems.

__ I have difficulty falling asleep.

__ I feel grief or loss.

__ I am exhausted by daily demands at work & home.

__ I feel stuck in a rat race.

__ No matter how hard I try, I never feel caught up.

__ I feel burdened by financial obligations.

28

__ I am under strain at work.

__ I feel lonely and unloved.

__ I am embarrassed to ask for assistance.

__ I feel overwhelmed by my responsibilities.

__ I can't stand criticism.

__ I'm afraid I'll lose my job or livelihood.

__ People let me down.

__ No matter what I achieve, I feel dissatisfied.

__ I stew in my anger rather than express it.

__ I feel apprehensive about the future.

__ My stress is caused by forces beyond my control.

__ I feel pressured by my commitments.

__ I have difficulty delegating.

__ I feel like running away.

__ My mind is churning and too busy.

_____ Total Score

- 0 to 18 = you are resilient and feel in charge of your life
- 19 to 37 = mild stress; with apprehension and some struggle
- 38 to 56 = moderate stress; feeling trapped, out of control
- 57 to 75 = high stress; life feels like one crisis after another

Chapter 3

The Importance of NERVE FORCE

Nerve Depletion

As previously noted, the millions of nerve cells that make up the vast Nervous System can be seen as reservoirs of nerve energy. The amount of nerve energy we store represents our entire precious Nerve Capital.

It is evident that if our nerve reservoirs are but 50% full of nerve energy – that is, half depleted – our nerve pressure will be half of what it should be. Thus our vital organs and muscles will receive only a fraction of the supply of Nerve Force necessary to enable them to perform their full duty, which is running the entire body.

Our nerve pressure is at its greatest height when our nerve cells are full of stored energy. We are then fully alive with physical and mental energy. No task seems too great, no strain too severe. We crave ways of letting off steam. That's when you become a human dynamo. You have double the energy and vitality of the average person! You have so much Nerve Force in your reservoir you are absolutely tireless! This is what my father and I have been able to attain for ourselves – and we want the same for you and for everyone! It's to be treasured and guarded.

As mentioned earlier, my father has been through the experience of extreme nerve depletion. There is no part of exhaustion that we cannot understand. Depletion and abuse of the nervous system leads to a motley group of organic, mental and physical weaknesses and disorders. The proper functioning of every muscle and every organ – in fact, every cell of the human body – depends directly upon the nerves for the initial impulse of life and power. It's inevitable that nerve depletion generally weakens the body and disturbs its proper functions – causing upsets.

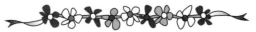

Our best preparation for tomorrow is the proper use of today!

29

It is not inevitable, however, that your Nerve Force must remain depleted. You can rebuild it! You don't have to drag yourself around fatigued and only half-alive! Mother Nature intended you to be full of vitality and nervous energy – regardless of your age! Follow The Bragg Healthy Lifestyle presented in this book and you will fill and maintain your reservoir with dynamic Nerve Force!

Nerve Depression

Nerve Depression means the shutting off of the nerve flow from the reservoirs, just as you would stop the water flow in a garden hose by stepping on it. No matter how full of energy your nerve reservoirs may be, your vital organs may be prevented from getting their normal supply of Nerve Force because of Nerve Depression.

The difference between Nerve Depletion and Nerve Depression is that the former can be a deep-seated general Nervous System weakness, whereas any Nerve Depression may be of a temporary nature. For instance, worry and grief can cause extreme Nerve Depression, which may result in death within a short time. The expression "died of a broken heart" can literally be true, because in some cases the heart is actually paralyzed by emotional distress! Nerve Depression has a direct and powerful paralyzing effect upon all the vital organs. A person who claims to be "worried to death" may be uttering a fatal truth! Worry can be a destroyer of health, youthfulness and life itself! (see web: *www.nmisp.org/*)

Yet, we all have to face worries at times in our lives. You can't escape them. If you have the physical and mental nervous energy required, you can face almost any worry without letting it harm and tear you apart! A full reservoir of Nerve Force lets you take worries in stride!

Beware of Computer Use and Depression: *A recent study found that healthy teens who used the computer obsessively spending 31 hours a week or more on the computer were more impulsive and less comfortable with other children; prone to suffer from depression; anxiety; drop in grades and sadly have worse relationships with their parents. It is clear Web Surfing and Gaming can lead to home, school and mental health problems. –* The Journal of Pediatrics (www.jpeds.com)

Of all the knowledge, that most worth having is the knowledge about health! The first requisite of a good life is to be a healthy person. – Herbert Spencer

Nerve Tension

Nerve Tension, stress and strain are caused by undue nervous excitement which produces over-activity of the nervous system, such as great fear and anger. It can even cause instant death. During the Great Depression of the early 1930s, Dad personally saw businessmen die from the tension, stress and strain of being financially ruined.

Under high Nerve Tension, a large volume of Nerve Force is poured out in a short space of time, thus causing extreme agitation of the vital organs. We have all observed that when we are angry or frightened our heart beats wildly, we breathe rapidly and our abdominal organs are topsy-turvy, sometimes causing sudden evacuation of the bowels or even some vomiting and the shakes.

Recognizing and Avoiding Hypertension

American Medical Association research indicates that people who have uncontrolled hypertension (high blood pressure) are more likely to develop coronary heart disease. They are six times more likely to develop congestive heart failure, and seven times more likely to have a stroke.

In the important Framingham Heart Study, doctors found hypertension responsible for 40% of congestive heart failure in men, and 60% in women. Hypertension was diagnosed in 91% of participants with congestive heart failure. The risk of developing congestive heart failure was twice as high in men, and three times as high in women, whose blood pressure was higher than normal (120/70) levels. Less than one quarter of the men and less than one third of the women lived more than 5 years after being diagnosed with congestive heart failure. See website: *www.nhlbi.nih.gov/about/framingham*

Your blood vessels can be severely damaged by high blood pressure. The force of blood pushing hard through your arteries can shear and tear off cells from the inside lining; this leads to a build up of bulging plaque, made of fat, cholesterol and dead cells. Those with elevated blood cholesterol levels – especially "bad cholesterol" (low density lipoprotein, LDL) are at greater heart risk for developing fatty plaques. (See Healthy Heart Habits, page 128.)

Hypertension accelerates the process, and the plaques can grow and eventually block the passage of blood – known as atherosclerosis – which can even begin as early as childhood! Like hypertension, atherosclerosis is silent until there has been enough damage done to cause symptoms. Nearly 1 in 5 with silent atherosclerosis have a heart attack as their initial symptom.*

High blood pressure can also speed up the hardening of the arteries – arteriosclerosis. This occurs when the muscles in your blood vessels become thickened and hard, which narrows the arteries and makes them less flexible. Therefore, less blood passes through the vessels to the tissues, resulting in coronary artery disease.

An EKG – electrocardiogram – can determine whether your heart is damaged or enlarged. An EKG monitors your heart's electrical activity. Your doctor may also recommend an echocardiogram, to evaluate and see the size of your heart and how well it is functioning.

Not surprisingly, physically active people are much less apt to have high blood pressure than sedentary "couch potatoes". Your diet can also affect your blood pressure. Eating low or nonfat foods, fresh fruits and vegetables and whole-grain foods, can help lower your blood pressure. Eating excessive amounts of saturated fat will raise the level of cholesterol in your blood. This can lead to increased chances of heart disease as well as developing cancer, diabetes and other illnesses.

Calculating cholesterol and fat is unnecessary – just avoid animal foods which are the main source of harmful cholesterol (LDL). It's best to avoid foods that had a face. The "good" cholesterol (HDL) high density lipoprotein, is formed only in your body. The] cholesterol is a larger particle that helps to remove fat from the blood and the artery walls. The Bragg Healthy Lifestyle with energy powered organic fruits, vegetables, whole grains, etc, a diet low in saturated fats, and getting plenty of exercise will help you avoid heart disease, hypertension and other life-threatening illnesses.

---

* Read the Bragg Healthy Heart Book to build a strong heart and prevent heart disease, strokes and heart attacks – the #1 killer of Americans. (See back pages for Bragg booklist.)

High Blood Pressure in Adolescence

Childhood obesity is particularly troubling because the extra pounds often start kids on the path to health problems that were once confined to adults, such as high blood pressure, diabetes, and high cholesterol. This research strongly suggests overweight prevention may need to begin even before the first day of school, promoting good nutrition, as well as exercise and fitness.

In the last two decades, the prevalence of overweight children ages 6-11 has doubled and tripled for American teenagers. The annual National Health and Nutrition Examination Survey done by the Center for Disease Control and Prevention found that about one-third of U.S. children are overweight or at risk of becoming overweight. In total, about 25 million U.S. children and adolescents are overweight or nearly overweight!

According to Mayo Clinic the incidence of childhood obesity is rapidly rising throughout the world. It is especially evident in U.S. where many children live sedentary lives – watching television, playing video and web games, etc. and eating more convenience fast foods, junk foods and sweets, which are typically higher in fat calories and low in healthy nutritional values. See web: *mayoclinic.com*.

Lower Your Blood Pressure Naturally

A government-sponsored Joint National Committee on Detection, Evaluation and Treatment of High Blood Pressure has been calling for a healthy (non-drug) lifestyle as a treatment for individuals with various forms of hypertension. Sadly over a third of Americans (1 in 3) have high blood pressure or hypertension.

News on High Blood Pressure & Diet

Researchers from New York Presbyterian Hospital have found that the mineral components of diets can significantly lower blood pressure, especially if one is suffering from hypertension. The specific minerals were potassium, magnesium and calcium (try Bragg's Apple Cider Vinegar for its healthy potassium). Eating a low-fat diet aids in lowering HBP and cholesterol levels.

Cardiovascular disease kills one Australian nearly every ten minutes! accounting for 34% of all deaths in Australia. (Compared to one victim every 34 seconds in U.S.) Sadly, many of these deaths were preventable.

Researchers examined 400 airport traffic controllers, who work under stressful high-pressure conditions. After a three year period, the air traffic controllers developed hypertension at a rate of three to four times higher than the normal population. Other research indicated individuals who move from rural towns to the big city, have an increase of blood pressure. Stress can result in significant elevations in blood pressure; this can overwhelm your cardiovascular system and make you a prime heart attack, stroke and illness candidate.

More than two decades of research in biofeedback have demonstrated that we can bring many Autonomic Nervous System (ANS) (see page 1) functions under our control if information about how to do so is made available. As we practice and identify what we're doing, figuring out what works and what doesn't, we learn to improve our skills – like learning to drive a car. Obtaining biofeedback (that monitors your heart rate and skin temperature) can aid in developing sensitivity and ability to modify your internal physiology towards better health.

Dr. Barbara Brown in her book *Stress and the Art of Biofeedback (amazon.com)* states, "When the mind receives information about itself, its body, how it reacts to stress and how it can return to well-being and then mental faculties of awareness and understanding are roused to action! By some obscure capacity, cognitive faculties are set in motion to restore the mind and body to a state of balance and relieve the effects of stress." By learning correct breathing techniques (read *Bragg Super Power Breathing* Book, pages 211-213), and muscular relaxation and imagery, the mind learns a new mental and emotional response. This eventually will result in modifications of the vital hypothalamus and limbic system – a specialized area within the subcortical brain, often referred to as the emotional brain. With practice, you can establish the voluntary control of the unconscious process and bridge the gap between the conscious and the unconscious.

Danish researchers found that with every 8.8 pounds of weight gain, the risk of developing ischemic heart disease increases by more than 50%! Ischemic heart disease is caused by a narrowing of the heart arteries, which reduces blood flow and oxygen and can lead to heart failure.

Prevention is always wisest and preferable to the cure!

Biofeedback Empowers You to Relax

A controlled study by Dr. Keith Sedlacek divided hypertensive patients into two groups. One group learned simple relaxation techniques accompanied by a bio-feedback method; the other received only medication. After a four month period, blood pressure had decreased in the relaxation/biofeedback group from an average of 144/95 to 120/70. Visit the biofeedback web: *brain-trainer.com*. In contrast, the medication-only group showed no significant decline in blood pressure over the four months. These antihypertensive drugs are not only costly, but often have unpleasant side effects which may increase the risk of cardiovascular disease. Therefore, a "step zero" approach is recommended – medication is gradually reduced, then eliminated to "zero" for the individuals who can regain control of their blood pressure through non-pharmacological, healthy lifestyle methods.

CIP – Constant Instant Practice is a process that rapidly re-establishes equilibrium in just a few moments and helps break the stress cycle naturally at its source.

This CIP includes 3 steps: • deepening your breathing • relaxing your muscles • warming your hands and feet

The instant you detect stress, extend and deepen your breath – for uninterrupted, smooth, even breathing are keys to stress control. Relaxing the muscles, especially around your shoulders, back and jaw counters your body's tendency to tighten under stress. Warming your hands and feet will decrease sympathetic nervous system activity. Your hands and feet play a critical role in your response to stress. While your body temperature varies no more than a few degrees from 98.6, the temperature of your hands and feet can vary nearly 25 degrees. If you're calm and relaxed, your hands and feet will become warmer. Warming your hands and feet (in hot vinegar water) calms the nerves and helps increase circulation that also helps normalize the blood pressure.

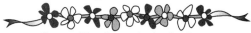

Breathing is our connection to life, through the body and heart, leading us to a wholeness of being and giving us spirit for living life to its fullest. – S. Hainer, M.S.

Self-Pity is a Nerve and Energy Robber

Another demon that you must dissipate is self-pity. Feeling sorry for yourself is a complete waste of energy. It blocks sympathy and help from others! When sorrow comes your way – face it and know that time will bring relief. Never accept despair or defeat! Remember that it is never too late to give yourself a second chance!

Above all, do not live in the past! That is all water under the bridge. The past has given all of us bruises, bumps, knocks, heartaches and torment mixed with joy. But there is nothing we can do about the past except learn some wise lessons. It's part of growing and maturing. Yes, many unpleasant things happen in our past. Remember, it wasn't all bad! There are a lot of bright, happy spots in everyone's past and those are the ones to recall!

Even if your past was a very happy one, don't try to live in it. Life does not run backward! Energy – a principle of Mother Nature – only moves forward! We cannot use it for ourselves in any way that is contrary to its laws. We cannot expect to hold energy, which moves forward, if we are thinking backward. Our energy depends upon our Nerve Force. That's why we must build powerful Nerve Force that will enable us to create health and happiness in all phases of our life!

Talk, Even Write to Yourself: You Can Be Your Best Therapist!

Kenneth Pelletier, Ph.D., an authority on stress, states that individuals who manage stress well – and even thrive on it – have learned to create "regular islands of peace" in their daily lives. You can achieve this by regularly taking brief moments of relaxation that brings your body and mind back to a state of homeostasis (or peaceful balance), as well as by using the CIP method.

Constructive self-talk and mental rehearsal can also help you to manage stress more effectively – for example, developing statements to say to yourself during times of stress. This internal dialogue along with CIP method will assist you in getting your body and mind into balance.

Negative thoughts influence our health! Studies show negative brain activity could be linked to a weakened immune system. – mayoclinic.com.

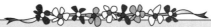

POSITIVE STATEMENTS TO USE:

- I listen to my inner self – I can do it!
- Feeling stressed is not going to help this situation.
- I'll just get started and then I'll be all right.
- Take things one step at a time, then everything will go smoother.
- Relax, be calm, plan, plot, and follow through.
- Problems are an opportunity to engage in solutions.
- I've done this before and I can do it again!
- Just take it easy . . . one step at a time.
- Try to think, hear or see things from the other person's point of view.
- The harder things get, the more dedicated I am.
- It takes two to have a conflict. I'm not going to participate in something that's not important and that will put more unwanted stress on me!

Create some of your own constructive, positive stress-management phrases. Write them on an index card and place them in your home, office and car. Make them part of your everyday positive thought process. Mentally rehearse – see, hear and feel yourself successfully responding to and managing any stressful situation which may arise. You can create new neurogenic circuits for healthier behavior patterns by imagining positive ways you wish to handle stressful circumstances!

Maximize Benefits of Positive Affirmations

Your happiness and your success in life is determined by the thoughts you hold. By consistently repeating positive affirmations you reinforce the new positive inner image you have of yourself. Let yourself really feel them. To maximize the benefits – use positive affirmations every day for at least 30 days. Also stop thinking negatively and replace with your favorite positive affirmations. See informative web for more examples of positive affirmations: *www.vitalaffirmations.com*

Some of life's greatest pleasures happen when we slow down, and enjoy the little things that brighten our life. – MacAnderson.com

I give thanks daily for all the Miracle Blessings I receive. – Patricia Bragg, N.D., Ph.D.

Some Need Professional Help

If you are frequently irritated, angry, anxious, severely depressed, bitter or burned out and are unable to resolve your problems, it may be advisable to work with a competent therapist. You might have to interview a few to find the right match. Call several and say you are seeking a therapist – could you drop in and say hello – then look, talk and feel if it's the right therapist. Even Hollywood Stars have wise advisers to converse with, and work out the roller coaster problems they often face.

Nerve Force is Powerful and So Important

Nervous tension, stress and strain can cause an excessive expenditure of Nerve Force. That is why we feel "drained" after a sudden fright, upset or great anger. Under these conditions even people whose nerve reservoirs are depleted to the lowest level can – for a short period – pour out an enormous quantity of nerve energy that produces unusual strength and adrenaline. For example, someone who is involved in an accident or emergency. This is particularly true of overly disturbed emotional people (*as 9/11/01 terrorists*) and also insane people.

We once read a newspaper account of 2 young boys, both only 14 years old, who were hiking in the forest when suddenly a thunder storm appeared. Lightning struck a tree which fell on one of the boys, pinning him down. He screamed in pain and fright. The other boy – exerting superhuman strength granted by his Nerve Force – lifted the heavy tree off his friend, put him on his back and ran for 5 miles to get help. The next day, the injured boys parents and several men went to the accident scene. Four adult men could not lift the tree! *A miracle for sure!*

We do not want to wait for such an emergency to drain our vital powerful Nerve Force from our reservoirs or to prove that we can exert it. We want to develop powerful Nerve Force that will keep our reservoirs full, as well as be aware of the fact that we have it.

38

Develop healthy self-esteem to generate positive lifestyle habits that promote more serenity, peace and love in your life. – Patricia Bragg, N.D., Ph.D.

Take time to do something healthy for yourself. Improving your outlook on life goes a long way in improving your health. Take care of yourself naturally and positively. – A Bragg Friend – Dr. Bob Martin, Secret Nerve Cures

Physical and Mental Deterioration

When your Nerve Force becomes depleted, you feel mentally and physically fatigued and exert yourselves only by utmost stimulation of your will power. In doing this you put draining stress, strain and tension upon yourselves. It is then that you try to fight your fatigue with unhealthy stimulants such as tea, coffee, alcohol and "Pep Pills", or drugs that will further exhaust your nerves as you head towards a complete nervous breakdown!

It is then that we begin to feel ourselves getting old, although we may still be young. A more pronounced decline is seen in our physical, mental and organic forces as our Nerve Force becomes more depleted. We lose our sex drive and the sparkle fades from our eyes. We lose the spring in our step and we lose our skin and muscle tone. Because of the sluggishness of our vital organs, we may begin to excessively gain or lose weight. We are then headed for the human scrap heap!

39

Impaired Metabolism Causes Body Imbalance

Nerve exhaustion seriously impairs a basic process of the body known as the Metabolism. This is the process by which nutritive material is transformed into living tissue (constructive), or living tissue and nutrients are broken down and used to produce energy (destructive). Every cell in the body is constantly engaged in either the constructive or destructive process, and every vital organ is a part of the intricate machinery of Metabolism. It is the life process, the basis of all health and all vital power.

When nerves are normal, there's a balanced harmony between the constructive and destructive processes of Metabolism. When this precious Nerve Force is depleted or exhausted the natural, healthy equilibrium is thrown off balance and the most noticeable results are excessive loss or gain of weight and lack of energy! (See page 175.)

A healthy diet, therefore, cannot be gauged in mere calories. We must eat the kind of foods that will help build our Nerve Force! This way there will be sufficient nerve energy to convert the food into tissue and then into energy to maintain a healthy balanced metabolism.

Post-Traumatic Stress Disorder

According to the National Institute of Mental Health (NIMH) nearly 7.7 million Americans have PTSD at any given time. Although more men than women undergo "traumatic" events in their lifetime, more women develop PTSD. The symptoms of PTSD can range from mild to life-changing; from concerns to major depressive or panic disorders that can shatter a person's well-being and health. This can lead to intense phobias, paralyzing fear or feelings of helplessness and horror. Maintaining good physical health is a key to recovery.

Nervous Disorders Upset the Stomach

As stated before, the Sympathetic Nervous System governs the vital organs. The master branch of this system is referred to as the Pneumo-Gastric Nerve System, whose center is the solar plexus, or "abdominal brain", known in Yoga as our wise second brain. The pneumo-gastric nerve governs breathing and digestion, hence its name – pneumo (lung) and gastric (stomach). It is closely allied with the functioning of all the organs.

Sometimes even the slightest nervous upheaval can affect the pneumogastric nerve. We have all observed an uneasy feeling in the stomach when we worry, our solar plexus is affected, and sometimes the back. In cases of severe Nerve Strain, the stomach may rebel against your putting food in by throwing it up. When upset don't eat.

Millions Suffer From Nervous Indigestion

Nearly every form of indigestion, gastric and other abdominal troubles may be traced almost directly to a nervous disturbance or an abnormal condition of the pneumogastric nerve. This applies especially to the conditions usually grouped under "Nervous Indigestion". These are often too casually dismissed by most as temporary discomfort to be relieved by a quick drugstore remedy which merely postpones the future inevitable!

The indigestion conditions include fermentation, gas, heartburn, sour stomach, hyperacidity and stomach bloating, which often result in shortness of breath and pressure on the heart. These conditions can produce heart irregularity, palpitations and even heart failure.

Heartburn = Higher Risk for Cancer

According to a report in the *New England Journal of Medicine*, those with daily heartburn or indigestion have a higher risk of esophageal cancer, especially those who smoke, drink alcohol or caffeine and consume fatty foods and chocolate. The acid levels in your stomach soar, eventually causing an alteration of esophageal cells which can become malignant. (*See solution bottom of page.*)

University of Tennessee Researcher, Glenn Eisen, has cited recent studies indicating that heartburn or indigestion, clinically known as gastroesophageal reflux disease (GERD) – stomach acid which bubbles up into the esophagus – can be treated with diet and lifestyle changes. "If you need acid-reducing drugs more than once a week, you should see a doctor".

Frequent dilation and bloating of the stomach, due to gas formation very often leads to permanent dilation and the forming of "pockets" from which the food cannot drain. In these pockets a very serious condition – ulceration of the stomach – may begin. A prominent surgeon told us that many serious stomach disorders are the result of stomach ulceration.

It is evident that we should combat the first indication of Nervous Indigestion with the means at our command, and not seek fast, temporary relief. We must get at the cause. There are no shortcuts to health! You must earn your health and Nerve Force.

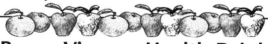

Bragg Vinegar Health Drink

A delicious, ideal pick-me-up at home, work, sports or gym. Perfect taken 3 times daily: upon arising, mid-am and mid-pm.
Recipe: 1 to 2 tsps Bragg Organic Vinegar and (optional) 1 to 2 tsps raw honey, 100% maple syrup, agave nectar, or if diabetic try Stevia (*4 drops or pinch of powder*) in 8 oz. glass distilled/purified water.

Bragg's Organic Raw Apple Cider Vinegar with the "Mother" is the #1 food I recommend to maintain the body's vital acid-alkaline balance. Also it's taken my Gerd patients off Tums and heartburn medications.
- Gabriel Cousens, M.D., Author of Conscious Eating

Do as I do – drink 3 Bragg Organic Apple Cider Vinegar Drinks daily.
- Julian Whitaker, M.D., Author of The Wellness Newsletter

Depression and Stress May Affect Diabetics and Cause Heart Attacks

According to Reuters Health Publication, a study has found that people with insulin-dependent diabetes who reported feeling depressed, anxious, or stressed out were among the least likely to successfully lower their blood sugar levels. The study found that persons with diabetes have the potential to benefit from realization-based therapies such as biofeedback, meditation and prayer.

Another study done by the National Institute on Ageing in Bethesda, MD, (*depression.com*) has found that when older men get depressed, heart attacks aren't far behind. They studied 3,701 people over 70 years of age, for six years. Among women, depression did not increase risk for heart attack or angina. However, among the men, the risk for heart attack or angina was almost double. When men are diagnosed with depression, it's important that they be closely evaluated for cardiovascular disease.

Other studies have shown that women are twice as likely as men to be diagnosed with clinical depression. According to researchers, the daily strains of work in and out of the home, coupled with feeling unappreciated by their partners and family, cause women to regularly think about their feelings. In turn, these thoughts feed stress. Women can help themselves by gaining greater control and solving their life problems, rather than dwelling on them. Also more education, achieving higher-level jobs and improving and enjoying work and home life are wise steps.

Nerve Depletion Promotes Constipation

Nerve depletion robs health and energy and promotes constipation. The action of the bowels depends as much upon nerve stimulation as the heart and lungs do. The bowels of a chronically constipated person will move freely when their nerves receive a violent shock, such as sudden fright, bad news or a violent emotional upset.

Diabetes is a modern, worldwide plague. Over 25.8 million people in U.S. suffer from it – 8.3% of the population. Even in China, Asia and Australia, diabetes is becoming a health problem as Western food makes its way into their diets. It is the major underlying cause of cardiovascular disease and kidney disease. Poor diets contribute greatly to this worldwide suffering. The greatest defense is a healthy diet, combined with exercise.

Refined foods, etc. increase constipation. In order to be entirely free of sluggish bowels, your food must contain fiber, moisture and lubrication. These important elements are found in organic raw fruits and coarse vegetables, such as celery, beets, broccoli, cabbage and carrots, etc.

Many people will tell you they cannot eat raw fruits and vegetables. This is because the Nerve Force in their stomach and intestines is at a low ebb and they don't have enough nervous energy to digest such foods. In fact, people on a bland diet often don't have the nervous energy to digest even the softest foods! That is the reason why so many people are nervous wrecks! They cannot digest any food, and therefore the nervous system, as well as the rest of the body suffers from malnutrition. We've met people who look like scarecrows, who are so low in Nerve Force that they are like literally starving to death! (Follow Healthy Heart Habits page 128)

For Easier-Flowing Bowel Movements:

It's natural to squat to have bowel movements. It opens up anal area more directly. When on toilet, putting feet up 6-8 inches on waste basket or footstool gives the same squatting effect. Now raise and stretch your hands above your head so that the transverse colon can empty completely with ease. It's vital to drink 8 glasses of distilled water daily! (pages 107, 128)

Feed Your Nerves – Don't Destroy Them!

Digestive and stomach trouble in extremely nervous people leads to a cycle of evils. First, nerve depletion impairs the power of the digestive organs. This creates toxic poisons which attack and further deplete the nerves. When nerve tissue is burned by toxic poisons, the nervous system can't function properly. Every victim that has indigestion problems, especially nervous indigestion, has observed that their nerves and health suffer correspondingly to the severity of the attack of indigestion. Few realize the beginning of the trouble lies in the weakness of their nerves (nerve exhaustion).

Eliminate the "Dribbles" Exercise: *To keep the bladder and sphincter muscles toned and tightened, urinate – stop – urinate – stop, 6 times, twice daily when voiding, especially after the age of 40. This simple exercise works wonders for men and women.*

Avoid Junk Foods and Harmful Stimulants That Cause Nerve Burnout & Health Problems

People with impaired nerves should use the greatest care in the selection of their food. Foods that continually cause indigestion should be entirely avoided. Many people who drink coffee, for example, will suffer from indigestion afterwards. The same is often true of rich pastries, ice cream, candy, cake, cookies, potato chips, hot dogs, greasy foods, hamburgers, ham, bacon, luncheon meats, mustard, catsup, pickles, and so many other devitalized foods. Many people also have severe stomach upsets from drinking alcoholic beverages.

Alcohol, tobacco and caffeine drinks like coffee, tea and colas are actually brutal whips that goad the nerves into action. Unfortunately, the nerves do not have the energy to obey for long. The drug caffeine stimulates the Central Nervous System and the coffee drinker gets a "lift" when the caffeine activates the nervous energy from the reserves. In time, this brings on nerve depletion and causes serious troubles within the Nervous System.

According to an analysis made by the Council of Pharmacy of the American Medical Association, an average cup of coffee contains about 150 mg. of caffeine. When you drink 6 cups of coffee a day, your system assimilates almost 1 gram of toxic caffeine!

Shocking Chart on Caffeine % Facts

Taking figures from the National Soft Drink Assoc. and the *Journal of American Diet*, you can compare the amount of (addicting) caffeine found in a 12 oz can of soda to familiar brewed drinks like coffee and tea:

SOFT DRINKS (12 oz)	Caffeine mgs	COFFEE, TEA (7 oz)	Caffeine mgs
Mountain Dew	55.0	Drip	115-175
Tab	46.8	Expresso	100
Coca Cola	45.6	Brewed	80-135
Diet Coke	45.6	Instant	65-100
Dr. Pepper	39.6	Decaf, brewed	3-4
Pepsi Cola	37.2	Decaf, instant	2-3
RC Cola	36.0	Tea, iced (12oz)	70
Diet Pepsi	35.4	Tea, brewed	40
7 Up	0	Tea, Instant	30
Root Beer	0	Matè	25-150

KEEP HEALTHY & YOUTHFUL BIOLOGICALLY WITH EXERCISE & GOOD NUTRITION

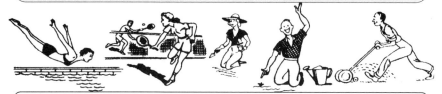

Always remember you have the following important reasons for following The Bragg Healthy Lifestyle:

- The ironclad laws of Mother Nature and God.
- Your common sense, which tells you that you are doing right.
- Your aim to make your health better and your life longer.
- Your resolve to prevent illness so that you may enjoy life.
- Make an art of healthy living; you will be youthful at any age.
- You will retain your faculties and be hale, hearty, active and useful far beyond the ordinary length of years.
- You will also possess superior mental and physical powers!

WANTED – For Robbing Health & Life

KILLER Saturated Fats	CHOKER Hydrogenated Fats
CLOGGER Salt	DEADEYED Devitalized Foods
DOPEY Caffeine	HARD WATER Inorganic Minerals
PLUGGER Frying Pan	JERKY Turbulent Emotions
DEATH-DEALER Drugs	CRAZY Alcohol
GREASY Overweight	SMOKEY Tobacco
HOGGY Overeating	LOAFER Laziness

What Wise Men Say

Wisdom does not show itself so much in precept as in life – a firmness of mind and mastery of the appetite. – Seneca

I saw few die of hunger – of eating, a hundred thousand. – Ben Franklin

Govern well thy appetite, lest Sin surprise thee, and her black attendant, Death. – Milton

Your health is your wealth. – Paul C. Bragg, ND, PhD.

Our prayers should be for a sound mind in a healthy body. – Juvenal

Health is a blessing that money cannot buy. – Izaak Walton

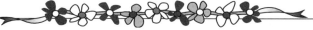

The natural healing force within us is the greatest force in getting well. – Hippocrates, Father of Medicine, 400 BC

Of all the knowledge, the one most worth having is knowledge about health! The first requisite of a good life is to be a healthy person. – Herbert Spencer

Mental Disorders

The physical pangs and ailments resulting from nerve depletion, great as they are, become insignificant when compared to the tortures of most mental disorders. The first symptom of mental instability is most often a lack of concentration power. Then usually follows the loss of memory, dizziness, melancholia, extreme irritability, hypersensitivity, suicidal tendencies and, at last, what is dreaded by most neurasthenics – insanity!

The Development of Neurasthenia

Neurasthenia is a neurotic condition characterized by worry, digestive and circulation disturbances that affects millions and creeps up without warning. Neurasthenia presents sinister danger to health and happiness and causes great misery. This ailment's development varies according to each individual's characteristics, but usually follows these stages:

First Stage

It begins with a lack of energy and endurance – "that tired feeling" or "the feeling that the body is made of lead" – making it an effort to move around. There is constant drowsiness and foggy thinking, a sluggishness of the vital organs and circulation, combined often with the feeling of extreme tension, stress and strain.

Second Stage

Here are some of the warning signs of nervous indigestion: belching, gas, sour stomach, heartburn, constipation, over-activity of the bladder, autointoxication (an extremely toxic condition) and biliousness. Breathing becomes shallow and difficult, with irregular heart action and palpitations. There is weakening of the eyesight, a decline in the sex drive, and a decrease in mental endurance and concentration. The neurasthenic is beset with dizziness, hypersensitivity, irritability, neuritis and other pains and sleepiness. There is a noticeable loss or gain in weight (due to impaired metabolism, as noted previously) and scores of other symptoms.

Third Stage

This extreme nervousness can often develop into nervous prostration, mental disturbances and also mental blackouts. An unbalanced emotional condition then ensues, often characterized by constant worry and melancholia. Serious body and mind disorders appear. Hallucinations develop, followed by suicidal tendencies and then insanity.

It is estimated that 95% of humankind has depleted Nerve Force to a greater or lesser degree. Look at the great number of cigarette users, for example. This is a destructive nervous habit. Most smokers are nervous and must do something to calm their ragged, stressed nerves. They get a false lift from the nicotine. It doesn't matter that nicotine is known to be a poison, or that warnings state cigarette smoking may produce lung cancer; the smoker has become addicted to their deadly poison and it's extremely difficult for them to break the habit (see page 136). The same holds true for other poisons that are used to whip exhausted nerves: tea, coffee, colas, sugars, alcohol and the harsher drugs. However, the law of compensation is at work on these people. You cannot get something for nothing! Most of these addicts will eventually have a complete nervous breakdown. As noted previously, 50% of the beds in all the hospitals in our country are filled by people with nervous and mental disorders and it's the world's #1 health problem today!

Millions Suffer From Nerve Exhaustion

How often do you hear of people going from doctor to doctor seeking relief for some mysterious malady or because "something's the matter" with them? Although repeated examinations fail to show that any organ is diseased or especially weak, these people persist seeking. The usual verdict of the physician is, *"There's nothing the matter with you, except you're a little run-down. You should go away and have a good rest."* In nearly every case, the real cause of this run-down unhealthy, toxic condition is Nerve Exhaustion, a very serious health problem!

In this age of strenuous living, the nerves are taxed so greatly that nearly everyone is a victim of some Nerve Exhaustion to a degree. The higher the state of mental faculties, the greater danger of nerve depletion. That is the reason why there are over 300,000 people committed to mental hospitals yearly in the U.S. There are also increasing numbers of uncontrollable and mentally challenged children who present grave problems to their parents and the educators of our country.

As discussed under Neurasthenia, mental illness is a condition which usually creeps up insidiously on its victim. There are many forms of nervousness. Each should be considered a warning sign to get busy at once, to build and restore the depleted Nerve Force. Moodiness is just one form of nervousness. Being "all keyed up" and unable to stop talking is another. Some people feel "all tied up". Others develop super-sensitive reactions, crying and going into emotional tantrums over the smallest matters. There are also those who become argumentative and aggressive, ready to fight and quarrel for no reason.

There is a long list of nervous conditions such as upset, nervous stomachs and headaches, sharp pains under the heart, heart palpitations and trembling hands and fingers. Some people lose interest in life and in everything and just sit around and brood. Others are overcome by waves of panic. They feel that something terrible is going to happen to them or one of their loved ones. Many people are overwhelmed by fears of all kinds.

AN OLD ENGLISH PRAYER

Give us Lord, a bit of sun,
a bit of work and a bit of fun.
Give us, in all struggle and sputter,
our daily whole grain bread and water.
Give us health, our keep to make
and a bit to spare for others' sake.
Give us too, a bit of song
and a tale and a book, to help us along.
Give us Lord, a chance to be
our goodly best for ourselves and others,
until we learn to live as sisters and brothers
in peace and harmony.

Chapter 4

Spiritual Health Promotes Physical Health

Meditation and Prayer

The First Step to Powerful Nerve Force

"Be still and know that I am God." It is in the peaceful silence of meditation and prayer that you find a higher power than yourself. This power can help, guide and direct you towards the healthy goals in life you are seeking.

It is important to set aside a period twice daily – morning and evening – during which time, the mind can go into meditation and prayer to build inner strength. There must be order and clear purpose to your thinking. Silently restate your new goals in life. Remember that you must displace the old, useless and damaging habits of thought with fine, bright, new healthy ideas.

49

Every constructive thought stimulates the nervous system with great vitality and vigor, and this sustained and powerful activity stimulates the entire body. Through meditation and prayer you are building a strong mind in a healthy strong body. You are building powerful Nerve Force because you are opening that inexhaustible reservoir of energy and creative intelligence which lies within each human.

Meditation and prayer will help establish equilibrium in mind, body and soul. It infuses you with new energy and expanded awareness, while it instills you with an inner calm and peace. You gain strength to do and to endure – to take the strains and pressures of life in stride. You will be better able to face whatever problems that may arise with sufficient Nerve Force to solve them.

Open my eyes, to behold wondrous things out of Thy law. – Psalms 119:18

Praise the Lord, our Savior! He carries us in His arms daily. – Psalms 68:20

Life is a precious, beautiful song and love is the music.

Simple Techniques of Meditation & Prayer

Meditation and prayer is powerful. It allows you to analyze your life in relation to your lifestyle, environment or with a particular person, thing, field of knowledge, principle, etc. In other words, you are getting yourself set for a glorious journey toward fulfilling your goals in life. You can proceed confidently knowing you have set yourself toward a destination or goal which you will achieve with lasting, rewarding success.

The Lord's blessing is our greatest wealth. – Proverbs 10:22

Ask, and it shall be given to you; seek, and you shall find; knock, and it shall be opened to you. – Matthew 7:7

Everyone has the capacity for meditation and prayer and it can change and empower your life! Only minutes of daily practice is necessary to reap God's lasting blessings. The effects of daily meditation and prayer for who you desire and want to be are blessings. Ask for it! You will notice benefits immediately. (Reread Matthew 7:7 and James 4:2.)

50

True meditation and prayer are completely free from mysticism and hypnotism. It offers you the ability to adjust to the fast pace of living with increased energy, self-confidence and greater peace of mind. It gives glowing inner happiness and brings harmony to the mental, physical and spiritual faculties. In turn, your reservoir of Nerve Force gets fuller, and stronger and your life becomes filled with daily miracles.

Daily meditation and prayer gives you the chance to strengthen your resolve to completely follow The Bragg Healthy Lifestyle. Your morning meditation and prayer allows you to plan your day constructively. Your evening meditation and prayer offers you the opportunity to review your day and evaluate your accomplishments and your mistakes as you plan how to correct the latter. During meditation and prayer, the body experiences a state of peaceful repose more profound than sleep. Studies have shown that the pulse, respiration and the metabolism slow down to levels below those ordinarily reached during sleep. People normally feel as refreshed following a session as they would after a nap.

No man can violate Nature's Laws and escape her penalties! – Julian Johnson

Meditation and Prayer Helps Master Life

Taking inventory of yourself this way is important. You will soon notice a much greater peace, tranquility and health within yourself. Life will flow more easily for you. Annoying events, things and people that used to bother you will no longer have the same effect upon you. This will give you more energy for creative thinking and living.

The release, peace and relaxation that is experienced following the meditation and prayer envelopes the entire day, with a softening effect upon your entire outlook and relations with life and others. The degree of personal involvement in emotional problems is diminished. This is not to say that emotional capacity is weakened! On the contrary, this wellspring is deepened as your inner life achieves greater life balance and stability. Meditation and prayer eliminates the causes of tension in a natural way (not like toxic tranquilizers), as it subtly sharpens the mind, heart and senses. This release from mental tension and physical duress gives a healthy effect on your entire well-being. Daily meditation and prayer helps to build a healthier balance to restore the body's normal rhythm of functions. Millions worldwide benefit from God's wise, practical and powerful guidance and love.

You Are What You Think and More

You will become immersed in patterns of decay if your mind is focused on negative thoughts and matters that are synonymous with disintegration. It's easy to observe the way this process works in the lives of others. It's much more difficult to see it in ourselves. Turn your mind away from negative thoughts, but not in distaste and revulsion. Rather, turn eagerly toward that which is new, fresh and desirable – remembering the wisdom gleaned from past lessons. Look ahead to the many years you will have to enjoy what and who you are, because of the experiences you are living through today. Waste no energy on recriminations or self-pity, instead move forward toward the bright future with new energy!

I cannot overstate the importance of the habit of quiet meditation and prayer for more health of the body, mind and spirit.
"In quietness shall be your strength." – Isaiah 30:15

Your Life is the Miracle of Miracles

You hold the miracle of miracles right now in the palm of your hand. You have the treasure of life! Think what that means to you! You are a living, breathing person! Life is the most priceless treasure on this earth. You have that treasure. Within you lies the mental power to be anything you want to be! You have a reasoning, logical mind. Within your being you have the kingdom of heaven. Find that heaven and you have reached bliss-consciousness. You'll have found heaven on earth and life becomes so precious and wonderful!

If you want more Nerve Force, energy and life, you will have to plan, plot and start creating, becoming and shaping your life! Look ahead. Have firm plans for living your life. Actually envision your future. You may change those plans and visions, but have them you must! Your creative force deep within you must reach out toward a bright future if you want to become one with the healthy flow of life! Your entire mind and being will be super energized in the process to go for your goals and dreams!

To Over-Rest is To Rust

Remember that your body will yield to your thoughts. **You are what you think!** By using your mind you sharpen its edge. Give it challenges with things to do and learn. Over-resting your mind gains nothing but its softening! Like the body, the more active you keep your mind, the better and sharper it will be. Recent studies show:

If you don't use it, you lose it!

To over-rest mentally or physically is to rust. Get the negative thoughts out of your mind and demand more action from it! Let nothing and no one stop you in your quest for inner mental strength, peace and happiness!

As you follow The Bragg Program for Building Healthy Powerful Nerve Force, you will feel the flow of new power surging throughout your entire body. Summon into action your will-power and self-determination! Faithfully adhere to and work on your new positive thoughts daily. Remember, flesh is dumb. Make your body obey your mind!

Build *"The Will to Win"* in Your Life
Life and Nerve Force flows through nerves at all times.

The more power you furnish to your nerves, the healthier and more well-balanced you will be. You'll get more out of life and have a greater chance of reaching the goals you wish to achieve! We all want to develop a strong mind in a strong body. We all want to be successful in life and reach our dreams and fulfill our life goals.

We'd like to share with you the ingredients of a winning philosophy. We've seen it proven in the successful people we have known. You've probably heard the phrase *"The Will to Win"* so many times that it has become a cliché, but stop and look at it afresh and realize its true significance. You must have this "Will to Win" if you are going to build powerful Nerve Force in your body. This is the indispensable first ingredient "Will to Win" in this healthy nerves and lifestyle program.

There's no better time to build your "Will to Win" than during your meditation and prayer periods. Tell yourself over and over that nothing and no one is going to stop you from building powerful Nerve Force! During your morning meditation and prayer tell yourself that you are not going to let anyone drain you of your emotional energy – no matter what they do.

53

If someone tries to irritate, nag or torment you, you are going to have the "Will to Win" over such circumstances. That "Will to Win" will keep you from stooping to another person's low level. Don't let anyone drag you down to their sorry level of emotional instability! It's not always possible to avoid people who are so miserable, unhappy and low in Nerve Force that they want to drag others down into the same state. Build your Nerve Force and make your "Will to Win" so strong that you will not be affected by these negative personalities!

To live is to know what counts and is important in your life. – Martin Grey

If you have been stricken by illness – your new car, your new home, your new big bank balance – all these fade into unimportance until you have regained your vigor and zest for living. – Peter Steincrohn, M.D., author

If you truly love Nature, you will find Beauty everywhere. – Vincent Van Gogh

You Need Inspiration To Guide Your Destiny

In every realm and arena of life, it is the person with a great "Will to Win" who makes their dreams come true. We talk about the human mind, the emotions and the body. We dare say that the most important thing within each of one of us is our will. Our own actions – guided by our willpower – are what ultimately decides our destiny.

Most people live life running in circles. They waste a lot of valuable Nerve Force going nowhere fast! If you are going to be a healthy, strong and well-balanced person, you must have a well planned and healthy sense of direction. You must know where you are going. Your inner compass will guide you in the right direction and be your inspiration. Yes, you've got to have inspiration! We wish we could tell you what inspiration was – then we would be the two greatest psychologists and philosophers the world has ever known!

54 Even people who rely most upon inspiration cannot tell you exactly what it is. Poets, artists and musicians can't tell you what inspiration is . . . but, we can all recognize its results! We have both seen total nervous and physical wrecks become suddenly inspired by a friend, health teacher, a book, etc. In a matter of months, they have rebuilt their minds and bodies and became healthy balanced people again. They accomplished what seemed impossible!

Although we cannot define inspiration, we would like to describe one facet of what we think it means when a person is inspired. It's when people clearly see themselves – not as they are – but as they can be. It's when they see themselves – not in terms of their weaknesses, poor health, low vitality, depleted Nerve Force and failures or the inadequacies – but in terms of what they want to become!

Faith and Vision Create Miracles

When you begin to believe you can be what your inner vision tells you that you can become – that's when you're inspired. When you no longer see your weaknesses – but your strengths – then you discover the power and ability to do things you never dreamed of doing before!

Health and cheerfulness naturally beget each other. – Joseph Addison

During your daily meditation and prayer you must forget your inadequacies and reach inside to find your strength – it's there! See yourself as who you want to be. Paint a vivid picture in your mind. Concentrate on that image in your meditation and prayer times and carry it with you daily. By following The Bragg Healthy Lifestyle, you are working with God and Mother Nature, powers higher than yourself! You are then living by inspiration, one of the most tremendous forces in this great universe! There is great truth in the Biblical statement that says:

> *They that wait upon the Lord*
> *shall renew their strength;*
> *They shall mount up with wings as eagles;*
> *They shall run, and not be weary;*
> *And they shall walk, and not faint.*

Those happy, healthy, strong and vigorous people – those people who accomplish greatness – all those of faith, possess a deep spiritual philosophy. They believe that their lives are protected by a Power greater than their own. They believe there is a destiny which guides their lives. **55** Nothing can thwart them! Following the Eternal Laws of God and Mother Nature they can accomplish great things!

Therapeutic Use of Forgiveness

Forgiveness sets us free from the past. Forgiveness is a process for most of us, wherein we work through grief, rage, sorrow, fear and confusion. Forgiveness comes at last as a relief and also a release for the heart. We can appreciate the truth that forgiveness is mostly for our own sake as a way to let go of any painful hurts and wrongs of the past.

Forgiveness is one of the great teachings we receive in our spiritual, mental and emotional life. Jesus so believed in forgiveness that he taught his disciples to forgive all their trespassers before they approached God's presence in worship. In Jesus' earthly ministry, forgiveness was often the operative word in both physical and mental healing. Truly *The Bible* is the main book of life and holds the treasures of how to live a healthy, peaceful life!

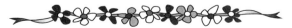

Count your blessings one by one and you will see what the Lord has done!
I give thanks for all the Miracle Blessings I receive daily. – Patricia Bragg, ND, PhD.

Let Mother Nature and God Inspire You!

We'd like to urge you to ask Mother Nature and God to inspire you in your prayer and meditations and, while following our Program of Building Powerful Nerve Force, to inspire you in your work, business and home. In God and Mother Nature you will find a power that will help you reach the heights of more healthy balanced living. Here are more great ingredients for a winning philosophy:

First: During meditations, dream great dreams and through meditation work to develop a will that translates those dreams into reality. Develop the *"Will to Win"*.

Second: Find inspiration in some great goal, some worthy cause or real challenge and let someone or something inspire you to see yourself not for what you are, but for what you can become and accomplish in life.

Third: Live by this Bragg Nerve Building Program, no matter what! Do the greatest good possible within you! Live up to the highest potential that you have! Accomplish those goals which have been set for you by God and Mother Nature! We know that if you meditate and pray twice to three times daily along these lines and build upon your inner strengths you will win, conquer and triumph with a long, happy, fruitful life!

The stress in our life can have mental, spiritual and physical effects upon us. One physical effect of stress is to negatively affect cholesterol synthesis, thus it can contribute to increased blockages in blood vessels. One way to handle stress is meditation and prayer therapy. This therapeutic use can take many forms and here are steps called "Prayer, Meditation and Forgiveness".

3 Steps – Prayer, Meditation & Forgiveness:

1. *Forgiveness from others. In your meditation and prayer time say to those who come to your mind you have upset, etc., "I ask for your forgiveness".*

2. *Forgiveness for those who have hurt or harmed you. In meditation and prayer, offer them your forgiveness.*

3. *Extend a full heartfelt, loving forgiveness to yourself.*

There Are Six Basic Fears

- Sickness • Poverty • Old Age
- Criticism • Loss of Love • Death

The majority of people – if asked what they fear the most – would reply, "I fear nothing". Their reply would be inaccurate, because every human being is, at some time, the victim of one or more of the six basic fears. Millions of people are crippled their entire lives by several or all of these fears. They live with high nervous tension while their Nerve Force is barely operating at a low ebb. Eventually, this causes a nervous breakdown.

Fear can attack the physical, mental, spiritual and material areas of life. It can strip you of your material possessions. In fact, fear makes difficult the tasks of procuring the bare necessities of life – food, shelter and clothing. Fear can destroy initiative, enthusiasm and ambition. It destroys your self-confidence and stifles the imagination. Fear can make you grouchy, dishonest, mean and irritable in your relationships with others!

Fear is dangerous because it generally exists in the subconscious and is not easily detected by its victim. If fear disclosed its presence by acute pain in the form of a headache, it would be less fatal. It would then be detected and its victims could eliminate it. Instead it comes like a thief in the night and poisons the mind so that it cannot function constructively for a healthy life.

You and only you can ferret out your fears and send them packing! No alibi will save you if you fail or refuse to rid yourself of fear because only one thing is required – the one thing that you control – your state of mind.

A strong state of mind is something that people acquire when they have built up large reserves of Nerve Force. Fearful thoughts are banished when there is powerful Nerve Force. This vital kind of Nerve Force cannot be purchased from any store – it must be created!

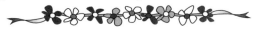

People with winning attitudes win!

With faith nothing is impossible. – Matthew 17:20

The greatest factor in pulling this country out of the doldrums of the great 1930's depression was the positive change in the minds of the American people in response to President Roosevelt's confident assurance,

"We have nothing to fear but fear itself".

A statement of timeless truth! Fear tends to paralyze. But if we face our fears intelligently, we can handle them.

Take a Hard Look at The Six Basic Fears:

Fear of Sickness

The seed of ill health lives in every human mind. To prevent this seed from blossoming into a terrible living fear, it is your duty to yourself to build your Nerve Force to its highest possible level. When the Nerve Force is very low, every ache and pain is magnified into a possible disease. The imagination runs wild. A person will have a headache and right away will imagine it's a brain tumor!

When you live The Bragg Healthy Lifestyle as outlined in this book, you'll banish the fear of ill health. There is a cause for sickness. You get unhealthy by unhealthy living! You are going to suffer from deficiencies when you eat devitalized, devitaminized and demineralized foods. If you're lazy, don't exercise – you lose muscle tone and get circulatory troubles, etc. Start living The Bragg Healthy Lifestyle and as Nerve Force builds, fears will vanish!

Fear of Poverty

There can be no compromise between poverty and riches! The roads to these two extremes travel in opposite directions. If you want riches, you must refuse to accept any circumstance that leads toward poverty. The word "riches" is used here in its broadest sense and refers not only to financial wealth but also to health, perpetual youthfulness, vitality, energy and long life – which are our physical, spiritual, mental and material estates. To us, the greatest true wealth is vigorous, vibrant health!

Fear of poverty is a state of mind brought on by nerve exhaustion. Build powerful Nerve Force and you will eliminate the fear of poverty. In fact, in the process of building powerful Nerve Force, you will already be traveling the Road to Health, which is your true wealth!

Fear of Old Age

When the Nerve Force drops to a low level, this great fear takes hold of the mind. It sends a cold shudder through the body of the worrier. They see themselves as old and feeble and a burden to everyone around them. They fear losing their eyesight, hearing, memory, hair and teeth and becoming weak, unattractive and senile.

This unreasonable fear of old age is one we all must fight by living The Bragg Healthy Lifestyle combined with constructive and positive thinking. Let us reason this "dilemma" out together logically and intelligently. First, there is no such thing as old age. There is not a cell in our bodies that is over 11 months old, except our bones and teeth. Every day we tear down millions of body cells and every day we build millions of new cells. So what part of us is old? The answer is – "No part of us is old"! The toxic poisons that get into our bodies, prematurely ageing us, are our main enemies – not our birthdays!

We hear this statement many times: "Man is as old as his arteries." That is definitely correct! There are many people 70, 80 and even 90 years old who have healthy flexible, clean and rust-free arteries. They have good circulation, keen eyesight and good hearing. They have learned how to keep their arteries free from clogging waste and toxic material. On the other hand, you find people in their 40s, 50s and 60s who have clogged arteries and suffer from premature ageing and health problems. Remember there are two kinds of ages – calendar years and biological years. The calendar years mean nothing if you live by the Laws of Mother Nature! We have friends who are over 100 years old by the calendar, but are leading a life that's superior to many people in their 40s and 50s. These people have found the *"Fountain of Youth* by living The Bragg Healthy Lifestyle!

Visit our web: bragg.com for more info on Bragg Healthy Lifestyle Living.

The true vocation of man is to find his way to himself. – Hesse

---

Most everyone turns to God when in anguish and in need.

---

*Optimism is the faith that leads to achievement;
nothing can be done without hope.*
– Helen Keller, famous author who was blind, mute and deaf.

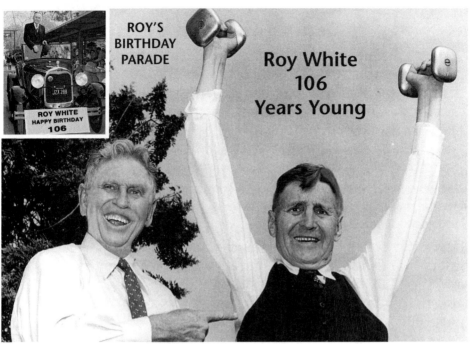

ROY'S BIRTHDAY PARADE

ROY WHITE HAPPY BIRTHDAY 106

Roy White
106
Years Young

Paul C. Bragg With His Youthful Friend
Their Love of Life Defies Time

60

My father's good friend, Roy White of Long Beach, California, is in his 106th year of life, yet he has a tireless, painless and ageless body. He knows the Laws of Mother Nature and God and he lives by them. He doesn't fear old age and is a young man in biological years. We both could name many, many more friends who are in their 80s, 90s and even over 100, who are biologically youthful!

A strong body and a bright, happy, serene countenance can only result from the fine admittance of thoughts of joy, goodwill & serenity into the mind.
– James Allen, philosopher and author, 1912

HEALTHY NERVE POWER: *For extra "nerve power" insurance, take daily high-stress B complex, and a multi vitamin-mineral with calcium and magnesium. Also, to relax and sleep better, try melatonin, magnesium, calcium & lemon balm (see page 74), Sleepytime herbal teas – natural relaxers that you can take before bedtime instead of sleeping pills.*

Exercise is the best natural anti-anxiety agent available. It reduces tension as it relieves aggression and frustration, aids concentration while alleviating distractibility, curbs the appetite and improves sleep.

It was Confucius who said: "Eat not for the pleasure thou mayest find therein; eat to increase thy strength, eat to preserve the life thou has received from Heaven."

Fear of Criticism

When the Nerve Force dips to a low level, one becomes extremely sensitive. Such a person feels that all eyes are upon them, ready to tear them apart with criticism. To eliminate this fear the first thing you must get into your mind is that many people are full of envy. The only way they can justify their own weakness is to constantly criticize others. Actually, such criticism is a left-handed compliment. It means that you are accomplishing something which the other person is not able to do.

A friend of ours who is a veteran of the political arena has often remarked, "If someone isn't shooting barbs at you, you aren't getting anywhere. The only time to worry is when you don't get any criticism – it means you're standing still." Always remember that no matter what or how well you do in this life you cannot please everyone – sometimes not even your closest blood relatives!

Dad remembers well those many years ago when some of his family and friends used to criticize him by calling him a "health nut," "food faddist," "health crank" and other more uncomplimentary names after he began to live in a healthy way. But Dad's Nerve Force was at a high level and they could not disturb his peace of mind. The long years have proved that my father's healthy lifestyle continues to build powerful Nerve Force, resulting in vigorous health and living in a state of agelessness. He had long since buried most of his critics!

Living by wisdom and intelligence, we let criticism pass over us like water off a duck's back. We live by the finer force of Mother Nature. We are one with God and Mother Nature. Therefore, why should we let weak, uninformed minds influence us? We are living at a high rate of mental, physical and spiritual vibration. When you live by truth and intelligence, petty criticism cannot touch you! You are impervious to slander and the talk of small minds.

61

Need a new hobby? Try volunteering at local homeless shelter, senior center, battered spouses or child sanctuary. Read for the blind or try helping with the disabled. – See web: www.dosomething.org

---

School seeks to get you ready for examinations; life gives the finals.

All that you do, do with Love. – Words of the Wise – Masada Lyrics

Fear of the Loss of Love

When your Nerve Force is at a low ebb, you are inclined to develop an inferiority complex and can easily lose your self-confidence. As you start to feel inferior you begin to fear that someone else may take away anyone who is near and dear to you. There is just one way to defeat this gnawing fear. You must build your Nerve Force so high by living the Bragg Healthy Lifestyle that any feeling of inferiority will leave you forever!

Jealousy is something all humans must fight. We can love someone, but that does not mean that we own that person. As you build your Nerve Force, you will see the wisdom of letting every person have their own personal ways. Build your Nerve Force so high that you will be above jealousy and the fear of losing your loved ones.

Love is the strongest force in the world! Give and be kind, understanding and loving, and you will be appreciated and loved more by family and friends. Remember that you can never lose one whom you loved and be thankful for the time you enjoyed and shared. With separations, hold no bitterness, as it can bring you unhappiness! You must remember that there are plenty of fickle people in the world and there is no use crying over their loss. In such cases, one might do well to remember this wise classic saying:

> *'Tis better to have loved and lost*
> *than never to have loved at all –*
> *Love is life's music that soothes the soul!*

The fear of being alone and unloved – although it haunts many people – is a groundless one. There is always someone who needs your love and who needs to love you. "Seek and ye shall find." All you need is the confidence that comes with health and a powerful Nerve Force!

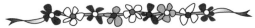

I know the sunny side of life. My Nerve Force gives me the power to radiate sunshine in the gloomiest of times. – Paul C. Bragg, N.D., Ph.D.

Every day the average heart, your best friend, beats 100,000 times and pumps 1,800 gallons of blood for nourishing your body. In 70 years that adds up to more than 360 million (faithful) heartbeats. Please be good to your heart and live The Bragg Healthy Lifestyle for a happy, long, healthy life!
– Patricia Bragg, N.D., Ph.D., Pioneer Health Crusader

Fear of Death

*It is not death that a man should fear, but he
should fear never beginning to live.* – Marcus Aurelius

> *Many die many times before their death.
> It seems most strange that one should fear death,
> seeing that death, a natural transition we all face,
> opens up to another realm for eternity –
> everlasting life will come when it will come.*

Accept death as a transition years away and then pass that thought out of your mind! Let youth and your years be a preparation for a wholesome, happy future and a fulfilled life! Then there is no reason why you should not die fulfilled after a long lifetime record! If you have worked well, done your share of good and service in the world, and have your affairs in order (your *will, trust, thank-you letters maybe with voice tapes*), then when heaven calls you will be prepared with a grateful heart.

We must all face and accept death when the time arrives. All life is a preparation for that grand climax for eternity. Govern yourself and affairs so that you can leave satisfied and hopefully, with few regrets! Live worthily so in time when you go to heaven you will be on God's honor roll!

63

Bear in mind that science has shown that the entire universe is made of mainly one thing – energy. It can be transformed, but it cannot be destroyed. Life is energy. If energy cannot be destroyed, life cannot be destroyed! Like other forms of energy, life may move through a variety of processes causing transition or change, but it remains as life energy. Death is merely a transformation. If death is not a simple change or transition, then nothing follows death except for an eternal and peaceful rest and sleep and is nothing to be feared! Thus, please rid yourself from the fear of death (*Read Psalm 23*).

Death is the furthest thing from our minds. We think in terms of living! Think like the Eskimos, who believe that as we fall asleep each night we die, only to begin an entirely fresh, new life when we wake each morning. We strive to make our days as perfect as possible!

Never fear, I go and prepare a place for you for eternity. – Psalm 23

Jesus spoke – I am the light of the world. He that followeth me shall not walk in darkness, but shall have the light of life and eternity. – John 8:12

The River of Thought

Life resembles a great river which splits into two different directions. One stream carries all who embark on it to inevitable success, health and happiness. The other fork of the river flows in the opposite direction, just as surely carrying those riding upon it to ill health, premature ageing, unhappiness and failure. This river is neither fantastic nor artificial. It exists absolutely as the Mississippi does, but in the minds of humans; it flows not with water, but with thought. The success fork of the river represents positive thought; the failure stream, negative thought. The most dangerous negative is fear!

Faith Versus Fear

Faith creates values. Fear destroys them. Faith builds! Fear tears down. It has been so since the dawn of civilization and it will be so until the end of time. All success has its beginning in faith. All failure has its beginning in fear. That is why we need to understand the nature and causes of fears and how to overcome them.

Fear need not be permanent. We can say this with confidence because we've learned first-hand about the uplifting power of faith versus the destructiveness of fear. The major portion of our lives has been spent helping people in all walks of life to master fear and develop faith. Innumerable times we have had people come into our offices or one of our Health Crusades so whipped by fear that they were ready to end it all by suicide! We have also seen these same people, after following our Nerve Building Program detailed in this book, change their lives with miracles and become ready, willing and eager to attack whatever problems life placed in their paths.

You cannot be free of nerve tensions, stresses and strains if you are full of fear. You cannot enjoy super health and youthfulness unless you have faith in God, Mother Nature and yourself! You must have such complete faith in Them and yourself that you can banish all of your mental and physical ills. When you build your reservoirs of Nerve Force through constructive healthy living, you can accomplish this goal of banishing fear from your life!

Overcoming Fears

After building your Nerve Force to the highest possible level you will be able to meet and defeat any of the fears that may come into your consciousness. We fully realize that it takes physical, mental, emotional and spiritual energy to overcome fear. Although you must face, confront and overcome your own fears, you are not alone in your battle! You can draw upon God's wisdom of the ages to help you.

New studies show millions of Americans use prayer daily that blesses their lives, and hospitals find prayer works miracles.

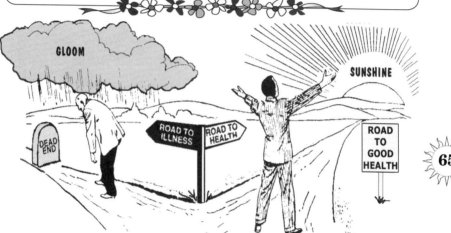

GLOOM

SUNSHINE

DEAD END

ROAD TO ILLNESS

ROAD TO HEALTH

ROAD TO GOOD HEALTH

65

NEGATIVE ⇦ OR ⇨ POSITIVE
The choice of which road to take is up to you.

You alone decide whether to reach a dead end or live a healthy lifestyle for a long, healthy, happy, active life. – Paul C. Bragg

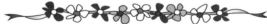

Eliminate the negative, latch onto the affirmative and accent the positive!

The secret of longevity is eating and living intelligently. – Gaylord Hauser

---

Deprivation of food at first brings a sensation of hunger, occasionally some nervous stimulation – but it also determines certain hidden miracle phenomena which are more important. The sugar of the liver and the fat of the sub-cutaneous deposits are mobilized, and used in order to maintain the blood, heart and brain in a normal condition. Fasting purifies our entire body and profoundly cleanses and modifies our tissues.
– Dr. Alexis Carrel, Nobel Prize Winner, Author of "Man, the Unknown"

The strongest principle of growth lies in the human choice. – George Elliot

---

Always do what is right – despite any public opinions.

Inspiring Words Bring Miracles

It is interesting to see how often one can find a source of spiritual energy to aid in the conquest of fear in both the Old and New Testaments of the Bible. Sign up on *www.crystalcathedral.com* for daily inspirational email. A few inspiring scriptures are listed here for you:

> *God is our refuge and our strength, a very present help in time of trouble, therefore, we will not fear. – Psalms*
>
> *The Lord is my light and my salvation; Whom shall I fear? The Lord is the strength of my life; Of whom shall I be afraid? – Psalms*
>
> *God hath not given us the spirit of fear; but of power, and of love, and a sound mind. – 2 Timothy 1:7*
>
> *There is no fear in love; but perfect love cast out fear. – 1 John 4:18*

Let a person lay hold of great words like these which come from those who have grappled with hardships. Let them repeat these spiritual affirmations during their meditations and prayers until their blazing faith has burned its way into their minds and kindled their own faith to best guide their thoughts, words and actions.

Along with The Bragg Healthy Lifestyle, you must look to a Higher Power for help to free yourself from fears, stresses, frustrations, strains and tensions. It's true – Man cannot live by bread alone! In your daily prayers you can meet with this supreme power and ask for guidance and then plan, plot and follow through for success in your life!

Don't flee from fear! Analyze it and see it as no more than a feeling. Don't be bluffed by feelings! There is an Eastern fable about a man who was being pursued by horrible dark shapes that he believed were demons. In a panic, he ran, desperately trying to escape his pursuers. At last, exhausted, he collapsed against the trunk of a tree and with wild eyes turned to face his imagined tormentors. "Destroy me!" he cried. "I can run no more!" To his amazement, the horrible shapes disappeared and evaporated like mist. They weren't demons at all, only fears of his own imagination that disintegrated when he turned the light of his eyes upon them and realized the truth! Read John 12:34-36, Psalms 119 and Matthew 11:4-6.

Chapter 5

Sound, Peaceful, Recharging Sleep

Second Step Towards Powerful Nerve Force

Sleep is one of the great Nerve Force builders. If you are going to have a glorious day, you must first have a splendid night of relaxed deep sleep. If you go to bed with a naturally relaxed and pleasantly tired body, a tranquil mind and a fairly empty stomach, you ought to sleep like a healthy baby! If you rise at dawn, give yourself the proper nourishment with natural foods and exercise vigorously in the open air, then you will surely be rewarded with sound, relaxing and refreshing sleep.

The person who is still tired and low in Nerve Force after 8 to 10 hours of sleep has usually not relaxed enough. Tense during the day, they remain unable to relax even in their sleep. Quality – not quantity – is what counts in sleep! Demand only the best and if you don't get it, ask yourself, "Why didn't I get enough sleep?"

67

Relaxed – Deep Sleep Must be Earned

It is impossible to get sound, relaxed sleep if you are constantly stimulating your nervous system with tobacco, coffee, tea, alcohol, sugar and cola drinks. A healthy diet of natural foods and correcting imbalances of body, mind and spirit are essential, as is open air exercise. Healthy children are physically active and the ones who play the hardest always sleep the soundest and get better grades. How can adults, who must cope with stresses, strains and tensions of modern life, expect sound, relaxed sleep when they don't get the required oxygen? If you want an excellent night's sleep, you have to earn it! You can't sit around all day eating, watching TV or working at a desk job with no exercise or outdoor activity and expect to get high quality sleep at night!

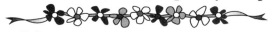

Help me Lord, to know the magic of rest,
relaxation and the restoring power of sleep.

Your Mattress is Your Best Sleeping Friend

You should sleep on a firm mattress or place a board under a soft one. This allows the muscles to stretch in natural relaxation and relieves pressure on vital organs.

CHECK YOUR MATTRESS

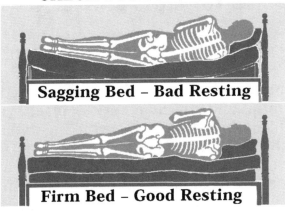

Sagging Bed – Bad Resting

Firm Bed – Good Resting

During our world health tours, we often have to move our mattresses onto the floor to be firmer. It seems that some of the world's top hotels put their money into showy lobbies and not into good firm mattresses. We also often find old, sagging mattresses in many of the homes we visit – but new cars in their garages! At our California desert home we had new wood platforms made. A firm mattress goes on top of this board with four legs on strong casters. Try a "miracle foam" mattress pad on top of the mattress – it's great. It might take you a few nights to become accustomed to being stretched out flat, but soon your body will thank you with more energy.

We travel all over the world in trains, planes, ships, buses, automobiles and often use soft foam ear plugs that shuts out unavoidable sounds and noises. We feel it's absolutely necessary that we sleep in a quiet place! Even though at times we do fall asleep when there is noise, the vibratory action of that noise can have a direct effect on the heart, circulation and nervous system.

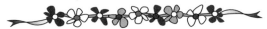

The average person spends about 23 years sleeping of a 75 year average lifespan.

Nervous Tension can ruin your health in many ways and diminish your productivity and shorten your life-span. – Dr. E. Jacobson, "You Must Relax"

We believe it's best to sleep alone. Two people sleeping in one bed is not as healthy because of body movement in sleep. Also, the toxins being released from another's body can be absorbed. Snoring (see page 77) and any restlessness of a sleeping partner are disturbing too. These disturbances can interfere with the other person's sleep. It has been proven by scientific research that a person gets a better night's rest and stores up more vitality when they sleep alone. Married couples will wake up more refreshed sleeping next to each other – each in their own twin bed. If this is not acceptable, then a king size bed is certainly preferable to the usual small double bed.

Dreams Can Reflect Past and Present Life

By exerting your willpower you can eat correctly, get enough exercise and breathe deeply – but you cannot sleep soundly by willpower alone. Through activity of the body and the brain you can cause weariness – but that will not insure you perfect rest. You may be too tired or too mentally excited to sleep. If you, for example, were watching a TV movie of violence, slaying characters and solving crimes you may find sleep reluctant. Don't waste time watching TV violence – it can cause restless sleep and even bad nightmares! But, when the brain and the body are moderately and wisely used, then sweet sleep follows.

However, too much sleep is often worse than too little! You can drug yourself with sleep to the point of stupidity, causing the blood circulation in the brain to become overactive and invoke frightening dreams. Fantasy can rise from the subconscious. Dreams can plunge you into the past, may even be at times distressful. Then with weary relief we wake to reality. Yet, isn't it strange? We have life's experience to draw on and dreams vary, reflecting experiences. It's healthy lifestyle living with sound sleep that lets us enjoy more life-changing, uplifting, peaceful, guiding dreams. *Web: www.sleeps.com*

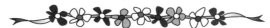

Motivation is when your dreams put on work clothes.

Read: "Dreams – Your Magic Mirror" by Elsie Sechrist, www.amazon.com

The sleep of the laboring man is earned and sweet. – Ecclesiastes

Books Can Be Your Teachers & Relaxers

Govern yourself so that your sleep will be relaxed and sound. Your day should be active, including exercise, yet never fatiguing. Your last meal should be early and not heavy. Your mind should be reposed by a few hours of reading, studying or cheerful talk before bedtime.

Be wary of TV shows, movies, and videos that are promoting crime, violence and immoral unhealthy living, etc. Watching a war, western or crime story on TV puts your nerves so on edge you could have a bad night of rolling and tossing. A travel, music or classic program is fine for the evening's pleasure. Don't watch any violence – it's poison to the brain and hinders sound relaxing sleep!

A long, quiet evening at home is the best prelude to sound, relaxed sleep. Have a shelf laden with books close to your bed. Choose books consecrated to this task like the Bible, *In His Steps* by Charles Sheldon, *In Tune with the Infinite* by Ralph Waldo Trine, *Men Who Have Walked with God* by Sheldon Cheney. Also, *Stevenson's Letters, Montaigne's Essays, Pepys' Diary* – these are always reliable. *Walden* by Henry David Thoreau, *Don Quixote* by Miguel de Cervantes and *The Diary of a Nobody* by George Grossmith are all old friends, available night and day. Enjoy *Prayer of Jabez* by Wilkinson, *Mastery of Love* or *Four Agreements* by Don Miguel Ruiz and, also *Chicken Soup for the Soul* series – they are soul inspiring. This list could go on for pages according to your taste. Go to your local library and choose books that feed your mind, body and spirit with strength and inspiration.

This is why we write Bragg Books, to guide and inspire you.

The simple act of just opening one of these subtly hypnotic volumes and turning over the pages is often enough to encourage golden slumber. Soon you feel it prudent to turn off the light. The window is open and pillow nicely adjusted. You take 10 long, deep breaths in and out slowly and give a sigh of thankfulness, and then give a prayer, letting your thoughts rise towards the heavens.

When you sell a man a book you don't just sell him paper, ink and glue, you sell him a whole new life! There is heaven and earth in a real book. The real purpose of books is to inspire the mind to do its own thinking! – Christopher Morely

Outwitting Insomnia

If sleep be coy, you might try some simple device to woo it. A rational way is to invite sleep by imitating its rhythm. Put yourself in a position of slumber, relax absolutely and – with closed eyes – breathe in the steady rhythm of sound sleep. Shut the door of your mind as well as your eyes. If this fails, try counting up to a thousand at pulse-beat time, checking off the hundreds on your fingers. It's usually a safe bet that you will never reach the last fingers. Or lie flat on your back with arms relaxed along the sides. There is something calming about this relaxed position that produces deep sleep.

Natural Ways to Cure Insomnia

Having insomnia can leave you tired, irritable and moody; but this disruptive symptom can be cured naturally. Just follow these simple steps:

(1) Exercise! Too little exercise can lead to insomnia. Try walking for 20-30 minutes in the morning and do yoga, chi gong or body stretches for 20 minutes in the evening.

(2) Avoid animal proteins, sugars, refined processed foods, cola and soft drinks for these can cause sleep problems.

(3) Eliminate all caffeine from your diet and avoid using medicines that contain caffeine, such as Excedrin; stop caffeine for 30 days and see if your sleep improves. Take calcium and magnesium one hour before bedtime.

(4) An hour before bed soak in hot bath, add 1 cup vinegar.

(5) **Here's a natural recipe for a good night's sleep:** soak 20 almonds, 1 Tbsp poppy seeds, and 1 Tbsp pumpkin seeds in 2 cups purified water for 8 hours. (All three are rich in tryptophan, which increases brain's serotonin levels, helping to induce sleep.) After soaking, blend seeds in the water, with 1 tsp raw honey, 100% maple syrup or blackstrap molasses until smooth. Hour before sleep, warm 1 cup blended mixture over medium heat and drink it. Refrigerate the balance.

Never hurry, never worry, live with leisure, grace and care.
For it's plain that constant rushing, never gets you anywhere. – R. McCann

---

Nature never deceives us; it is always we who deceive ourselves. – Jean Rousseau

6 Hour before bed make cup herbal tea. Pour cup boiling water over 2 tsps dried valerian herb root, cover, steep 15 minutes. Strain, add raw honey or herb stevia (page 177) and drink. Or hour before bed take ½ to 1 tsp valerian extract in juice or 400 - 800 mgs valerian caps. Sleep experts say valerian is most effective for falling asleep faster and staying asleep longer. It calms the nervous system, relaxes muscles and acts like a sedative since the herb binds to amino acid receptors in the brain that are linked to anxiety. See webs: *www.sleepquest.com* and *www.naturalhealthmag.com*

Fitness Trainers Say Days Off Benefit Fitness

You don't expect fitness trainers to say a day off from exercise is good for you. However, the body does need time to rest and repair itself. Those who cut back to 3 to 4 times weekly got better results than daily exercise.

Food and Drink – Their Effects on Sleep

Drinking too much caffeine leaves most people very nervous and sleepless at night. However, other foods and eating habits can also contribute to restless slumber.

If you're having trouble sleeping, check this list:

1. Don't over-eat before bedtime. A large meal one or two hours before bed tends to keep you awake, and also puts on more weight. The body is then busy digesting food and isn't ready to shut down for the night.

2. Avoid eating heavy, high-fiber, gas producing foods late at night. Sometimes beans, nuts, raw onions and cabbage can cause some bloating and make sleep difficult. Eat them earlier to allow more digestion time. *Beano* helps.

3. Don't go to bed hungry. A light fruit snack (*apple, banana, grapes, pear, etc.*) will keep your brain from signaling hunger to the body at night that might wake you up.

4. No alcohol. It interferes with the deepest, most restful sleep states, and it also dehydrates the body.

5. Beware of all caffeine (some green teas have caffeine). It's wise to read labels before eating and drinking so you know what you are eating! (See pages 44, 101.)

A good laugh, a walk and a long sleep are the best cures in the doctor's book.

Simple Ways to Keep Stress Levels Low

❤ Keep a journal. Recording your feelings every day is an excellent way of getting them out of your system.

❤ Do some soul searching. Explore your unexamined self, through group therapy or a 12-step program.

❤ Meditate, pray or listen to soft music 4 to 6 times a day. These "healing times" will allow you to slow down.

❤ Live one hour at a time, paying close attention to your feelings. Allow them to surface, write them down, then take charge and resolve to release the wrong ones.

❤ Learn to love and protect your physical body. Don't waste time on negative energy! Examine negative thought messages you've been telling yourself all these years. Now change them by addressing your body with love.

Remember, your life is a series of moments where you are the captain. You are in charge! Make the most of them all!

67% American Adults are Sleep Deprived

A National Sleep Foundation poll taken recently discovered that 67% of American adults have sleeping problems. Shockingly they found over one-third (37%) are so sleepy during the daytime that their daily activities become difficult and often interfered with. See: *sleepdisorders.about.com* and *sleepfoundation.org* and for sleep disorder centers: *www.ninds.nih.gov.*

Over the past 100 years, we've reduced our average sleep time by 20% and, over the last 25 years, added an additional month to our annual work/commute time. Thus, our national "sleep debt" is rising and while our society has changed, our physical bodies and needs have not. We are paying a dear price for such "progress"!

Are You Getting Enough Sleep Lately?

The odds are you aren't getting sufficient sleep. American adults presently average 7 hours nightly. While everyone's sleep needs vary, most scientific research and studies indicate that we require 8 hours of sleep nightly.

Few are lucky enough to enjoy 5 to 6 hours of sleep and still perform well at work. To just get "caught-up", a full ten hours of rest is frequently needed and called for!

Try Lemon Balm Tea for a Night So Calm

First, make a clear and conscious choice about how you wish to spend the sixty minutes that precede your actual going to bed time. Avoid a rush to "get things ready for tomorrow" or to catch up on tasks not completed during the day. This is a time to relax and rest your body and mind. Try an aroma herbal bath or a self massage (*use Bragg Organic Olive Oil*) while showering, one hour before bed – it's so relaxing. Enjoy a warm soothing Bragg Apple Cider Vinegar drink with cinnamon and honey (recipe on page 41 & 114) or a soothing Lemon Balm or Sleepytime herbal tea hour before bedtime.

Lemon Balm, whose scientific name is *melissa officinalis*, is a cooling plant with both nervine and antiseptic relaxing qualities. It's a member of the Labiatae family, which also includes peppermint and spearmint, lemon balm is native to most areas of Europe and is now widely grown worldwide. Flowering between June and October, it's lemon-like fragrance is unmistakable and makes a delicious tea.

Like restful chamomile, lemon balm's primary, volatile oil makes the plant medicinal. While appearing to be just a simple plant, it delivers a wide range of potent aids for complaints ranging from stomach pain to the worst cases of insomnia. Try lemon balm tea after meals and before bed, miraculous results have been reported. Also, try blending with a variety of herbal teas. Some others to try for sound sleep are: sleepytime, skullcap, and valerian herbal teas, available health stores. Also try magnesium and calcium supplements and melatonin (1-3 mg) or its tea one hour before bed. Record results in Daily Journal (see page 110).

An effective herbal remedy for sleep is chamomile tea. Lavender and hibiscus teas are also very good sleep inductors. Also be cautious that you're not drinking tea which contains any type of stimulant or caffeine. For more info see: www.sleep-sense.com/102/tea-that-helps-you-sleep/

Avoid drinking too many liquids in the evening. Drinking lots of water, juice or tea may result in frequent bathroom trips throughout the night. Be careful of caffeinated drinks, which act as diuretics, that only make things worse. For more sleep info see: helpguide.org/life/sleep_tips.htm

Good Sleep is the Cornerstone of Health

Eight hours per night is the optimal amount of sleep for most adults. Science has established that a deficit of sleep can have serious, far reaching effects on your health!

Interrupted or Impaired Sleep Can:

- Dramatically weaken your immune system
- Accelerate tumor growth with severe sleep dysfunctions
- Cause a pre-diabetic state, making you feel hungry and can wreak havoc on your weight
- Seriously impair your memory. Even a single night of poor sleep (4-6 hours) can impact ability to think clearly
- Impair your performance on physical or mental tasks
- Can also increase stress-related disorders including: Heart Disease, Stomach Ulcers, Constipation, Mood Disorders, Personality Upsets and Depression

Healthful Tips for Sound, Recharging Sleep
Excerpts from Dr. Mercola – www.mercola.com

The good news is there are many natural techniques you can learn to restore your "sleep health". Whether you have difficulty falling asleep or feel inadequately rested when waking up, you can find relief from the tips below:

• **Sleep in complete darkness.** Even the tiniest bit of light in the room can disrupt your internal clock and your pineal gland's production of melatonin and serotonin. Little bits of light pass directly through your optic nerve to your hypothalamus, which controls your biological clock. Light signals your brain that it's time to wake up and starts preparing your body for ACTION!!!

• **Wear an eye mask to block out light.** It is not always easy to block out every stream of light using curtains or blinds.

• **Keep bedroom temperature lower (60-65°F is best for sleeping!).** Scientists state more cooler bedroom is conducive to sleep since it mimics body's natural temperature drop.

• **Check bedroom for Electro-Magnetic Fields (EMFs).** EMF's can disrupt the pineal gland and production of melatonin and serotonin. To do this you will need a gauss meter (Radio Shack sells them). Before bed unplug any phones, radios, etc. near bed, even when in hotels!

- **Turn off cell phones, move alarm clocks (battery-powered O.K.), computers, WiFi and other electric devices away from bed.** Lights, EMF's, etc. disturb sleep. Historically, people went to bed shortly after sundown, as most animals do, which is what nature intended for humans as well.

- **Get to bed as early as possible.** *"I enjoy early to bed, early to rise, keeps me healthy, happy and wise."* – PB

- **Establish a bedtime routine.** This could be meditation, deep breathing, aromatherapy, essential oils or a massage.

- **Don't drink fluids 1-2 hours before bedtime.** This helps reduce frequency of needing to get up to go to the bathroom. (Some like old-fashioned potty near bed.) **Also go to the bathroom right before you go to bed.**

- **Have a high-protein soy drink several hours before bed.** This can provide the L-tryptophan needed for your melatonin and serotonin production.

- **Avoid before-bed snacks, particularly grains & sugars.**

- **Take a hot bath, shower or sauna before bed.** The temperature drop from getting out of bath or shower gives signals to your body it's time for bed and recharging sleep.

- **Wear socks to bed.** Study shows wearing cotton or wool socks reduces night wakings. In winter fill Bragg Vinegar glass bottle with hot water, place at feet. It's a comfort!

- **Put work away at least one hour before bed.** This gives your mind a chance to unwind so you can go to sleep feeling calm, not hyped up or anxious about tomorrow's deadlines.

- **No late TV before bed,** disrupts pineal gland function.

- **Keep a Journal.** Do it in the morning when brain is functioning at its peak and cortisol levels are high.

For Relaxing Delights Try These:

SIGHT:	*Soften lights, close eyes & visualize beautiful nature scenes.*
SOUND:	*Soothing music increases the healing & reduces the stress hormone cortisol by 25%.*
SMELL:	*Aroma bath, use a few drops of essential oils. Try lemon, chamomile, lavender or sandalwood. These all have calming, relaxing effects.*
TASTE:	*During a bath savor fresh fruits or juices to replenish fluids.*
TOUCH:	*Get a massage or give yourself one in bath or shower. Lightly dab Bragg Olive Oil over body, massage feet, then neck, shoulders, arms and legs for relaxing health therapy.*

Lifestyle Suggestions That Enhance Sleep

- Avoid stimulants: caffeine (in coffee, some teas, even green teas, soft drinks, chocolate, sugar) and nicotine (found in cigarettes and other tobacco products).
- Don't drink alcohol to "help" you sleep, it's unhealthy!
- Have herbal teas – anise, lemon balm, Sleepytime, chamomile (beware some Green Teas have caffeine), or try melatonin, tryptophan (5HTP), valerian, calcium and magnesium supplements; they work miracles.
- Exercise regularly, but try to be finished with your workout no sooner than 2 hours prior to bedtime.
- Avoid foods you may be sensitive to. Reactions can cause excess congestion, gastrointestinal upset, bloating or gas.
- Associate your bed with recharging sleep – it's wise not to sit on it to work or watch TV. *Try a memory 2" foam topper (so comfortable) on your firm mattress.*
- If you suffer from insomnia, don't nap during the day. Remember, earn better sleep by exercise and day activity.

77

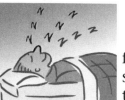

Relief for Snorer in the House

Now there are choices in treatment for relieving stubborn snoring. A simple doctor laser treatment, but first try the nasal strips (adhesive band-aid-like device) that helps keep open nose's nasal passages and allows easier airflow during sleep. Available at pharmacies, sizes small to large.

The second is RIPSNORE™. A simple, one-piece device that molds to the shape of your mouth. The device is very flexible when being fitted. It stops snoring or drastically reduces snoring in 98% of people who started using it. The RIPSNORE™ holds the lower jaw slightly forward, moving base of tongue away from back of the airway and soft palate - allowing throat to be opened and the snore to be silenced. The device is almost identical to dental ones, but is obviously a lot more affordable. See to order on web: *www.ripsnore.com.*

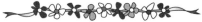

The Lord gives rest and strength to those who are weary. – Isaiah 40:29

A recharging, peaceful good night sleep is vitally important!

Stanford's Suggestions for Improving Sleep

According to Derek Loewy, Ph.D., Co-Director of the Stanford Sleep Disorders Clinic's Insomnia Program (*www.stanford.edu*), the first group therapy program for insomnia in the U.S., "Our insomniacs tend to be those with the thickest medical charts." Loewy suggests that if you don't fall asleep quickly, get out of bed and do something relaxing and enjoyable. He also advocates breathing exercises that promote relaxation and help patients deal with their sleep deficit. Loewy's program shuns drugs, "Although sedatives can induce sleep, they lose effectiveness as the body develops tolerance and addiction becomes a possibility." Here's more suggestions:

1. Have set times for waking up and also going to bed, it helps the body's sleep-wake cycle settle into a rhythm.

2. Stop caffeine, especially in afternoons and evenings.

3. Don't drink alcohol at night, it suppresses both deep sleep and dream sleep. It may allow you to fall asleep more easily, but you're likely to suffer a sleep disruption several hours later. Alcohol has many ill side-effects.

Remember sleep comes to the body when it's relaxed. When you lie down on your bed, let your body relax until you seem to sink down through the mattress and through the floor and beyond. Let go all muscular and mental tension – this is the secret of sound sleep!

The art of muscular relaxation should be practiced throughout the day. To understand the reason for this practice, note the furrowed brow of most business people, the tensely clasped hands of the nervous woman or the strained look of city dwellers. Everyone who is subjected to nervous tension, stress or strain – regardless of their occupation – should have periods for muscular relaxation during the day. If someone does fine work requiring constant use of their eyes, they should relax their eye muscles by looking away at distant objects. A writer should leave the computer to tidy the office or take a rest. Whatever your work, change your set of duties several times a day. Take a few moments at regular intervals to completely relax all the muscles of your body. Go limp, close your eyes and think pleasant, cheerful thoughts.

The Luxury of the Siesta

Spain, Switzerland, Mexico, France, Italy, South America and many others are highly advanced when it comes to relaxation. They have a rest period in the middle of the day. They eat their lunch, then lie down for deep, relaxing rest and sleep. Blessings and praises to the founders of this custom! This healthy custom – which years ago was prevalent throughout our own Southern States – has unfortunately become banished by modern Americans now. The abandonment of the afternoon nap is a high price to pay for so-called progress!

My father and I always have enjoyed our daily siesta – the "40 winks" after lunch. When we wake after our short after-lunch snooze, we feel that we're beginning a whole fresh new day! The midday siesta (30-60 minute snooze) gives you two days in one! It will recharge your batteries and send you back into the game of life with renewed vigor! If either one of us ever becomes President of the U.S., our first official proclamation would be, "A one and a half hour healthy midday break for all!"

Digestively speaking, your stomach requires what is known as the eupeptic pause after eating. For a short time after lunch and dinner, let your stomach have the center stage so your energy can fully concentrate on digesting the meal you just gave it. Allow the body to supply energy to your stomach as exclusively as possible.

Try Power Nap For Miracle Recharge

If you experience low energy levels around mid-afternoon, it's very typical for some. Many people are sleep-deprived which also adds to low energy levels. Even a 20-30 minute nap after work will leave you far more refreshed and alert for the evening than anything else. But avoid sleeping too long because you can run the risk of not being sleepy for your normal bedtime.

Healthy Mind Habit:

Wake up and say – Today I am going to be happier, healthier and wiser in my daily living! I am the captain of my life and am going to steer it to living a 100% healthy lifestyle! Fact is happy people look younger & have fewer health problems! – Patricia Bragg, ND, PhD., Pioneer Health Crusader

How to Have Deep, Sound, Relaxed Sleep

Let your sleeping tonic be composed of exercise in fresh air and sunshine. You do not get sound, healthy sleep when you take a sleeping drug – you simply get drugged! It is a vicious habit which may lead you toward a complete nervous breakdown. These drugs are both addictive and dangerous. As time goes on, habitual drug users must resort to increased dosages. These pills can – and do – kill!

Always keep in mind that tobacco, coffee, tea and cola drinks can cause sleeplessness! A heavy meal in the late evening can also give you a poor night's rest.

You should sleep on a firm mattress. This helps to stretch your muscles in natural relaxation. My father's bed is a wooden board with a firm mattress. What wonderful sleep you get when the muscles and bones of the body are held securely in place! Your sleeping space should be at lease 36 inches in width. If you have a sleeping partner, the bed should therefore be 72 inches wide or a queen or king size. But, in our personal opinion, for two people to share the same bed for sleeping purposes is unhealthy. To sleep well, it's best to sleep alone in your own bed. Couples do well with beds pushed together.

At the rate of eight hours of sleep per 24 hour period, we spend a third of our lives in bed. With this in mind, get yourself the best bed and bedding you can buy. Remember that its value is not necessarily determined by the sum you pay, but by the quality of restoring sleep it gives you!

Wear comfortable cotton or silk nightclothes, if any. There is a delicious freedom and freshness in sleeping naked, especially in the summertime.

A night of sound, peaceful, relaxing, refreshing and rejuvenating sleep is your finest health insurance! Woo sleep. Work to win it. Let it fill your body's reservoirs with powerful Nerve Force. Sleep is one of your best friends! Sleep is kind, it heals and recharges your Nerve Force.

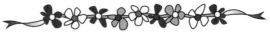

Lavender helps you relax. *Before drying off after your night bath or shower, place 3 drops of lavender essential oil on a damp washcloth and rub it gently over your body. The soothing active agents in the lavender oil will enter into your body through your skin and nose.*

Chapter 6

Natural Healthy Food

Third Step Towards Powerful Nerve Force

A happy life consists of tranquility of the mind. The instrument of the mind is the brain, which is part of the physical body. It's impossible to have this tranquility of the mind if the brain is suffering from malnutrition.

Most brains in our society today are undernourished. Never before in history have we had so many mentally challenged children! Never before have we had so many people suffering from mental disease! A traveler from outer space would look down on the earth and say, *"What a mess you have made of your beautiful planet!"*

You know the sick condition of this planet: the wars, terrorism, crimes, the starving millions, the hatreds and jealousies that turn nation against nation and man against man. Today, we live in a nervous, jittery world, a sick world that's getting sicker by the hour! Many young people take one look at this ugly, sick world and run straight to drugs to escape reality. Of course, no one can live without experiencing some degree of stress, strain and tension. There is almost no way of escaping these factors of modern living unless we find a fantastic dream island and live there in complete isolation.

What we must do is equip ourselves to withstand the effects of the pressures we encounter. To do this, we must build powerful Nerve Force. Our Central Nervous System – with the brain as its center – must be strengthened and kept healthy with proper nourishment. One of the most critical factors closely related to the health of the Central Nervous System is the B-Complex vitamins. When the body has an adequate amount of these nutrients, it can withstand the stress, strain and tension that our mile-a-minute life causes.

However, our modern "dead" foods are sadly lacking in this vital ingredient. Since the civilized diet has very little of the vital B-Complex vitamins, our bodies suffer from the same deficiency. No wonder the world is sick!

You need to learn not only what to leave out of your diet, but also, as importantly, what you should put into it. You will find that you can nourish your body without sacrificing meal-time enjoyment once you understand the basic health principles of proper nourishment. This knowledge will show you the elements your body needs to build, develop and live healthily as it was meant to do naturally. Combinations of healthful foods packed with vital nutrients are abundant worldwide.

The first step, of course, is to get into *the habit of eating for health*. Such a habit is not difficult to form. Although the instinctive sense of food selection has been submerged with all the advertising of the popular fast, junk foods, etc. You have to be strong minded! Like any other ability or skill, a healthy lifestyle must be kept constantly in practice or its powers will deteriorate. Only by exercising this natural health instinct and desire can we revive and strengthen our health.

82

Bad Nutrition –
#1 Cause of Sickness
"Diet-related diseases account for 68% of all deaths."
– Dr. C. Everett Koop

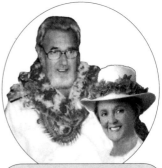

Dr. Koop & Patricia

Hawaii Health Conference

America's former Surgeon General and our friend, said this in his famous 1988 landmark report on nutrition and health in America. People don't die of infectious conditions as such, but of malnutrition that allows the germs to get a foothold in sickly bodies. Also, bad nutrition is usually the cause of non-infectious, fatal or degenerative conditions. When the body has its full nutrition quota of vitamin and minerals, including potassium, it's almost impossible for germs to get a foothold in a healthy, powerful bloodstream and tissues!

Junk foods, processed meats, hot dogs, sausage, sugar and fast foods can increase inflammation in your body which could lead to chronic disease.
– Dr. Bob Martin, author Secret Nerve Cures • www.doctorbob.com

What a person eats becomes his own body chemistry.

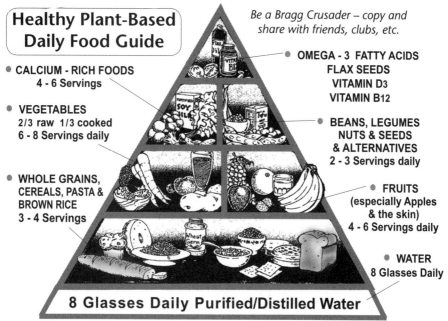

Healthy Plant-Based Daily Food Guide

Be a Bragg Crusader – copy and share with friends, clubs, etc.

- **OMEGA - 3 FATTY ACIDS**
  FLAX SEEDS
  VITAMIN D3
  VITAMIN B12

- **CALCIUM - RICH FOODS**
  4 - 6 Servings

- **VEGETABLES**
  2/3 raw 1/3 cooked
  6 - 8 Servings daily

- **BEANS, LEGUMES NUTS & SEEDS & ALTERNATIVES**
  2 - 3 Servings daily

- **WHOLE GRAINS, CEREALS, PASTA & BROWN RICE**
  3 - 4 Servings

- **FRUITS**
  (especially Apples & the skin)
  4 - 6 Servings daily

- **WATER**
  8 Glasses Daily

8 Glasses Daily Purified/Distilled Water

The above Food Guide Pyramid illustration represents a more ideal way of eating for achieving optimal nutrition, health and wellness. You will notice that this Food Guide Pyramid is based on healthy organic plant foods, with emphasis on pure water, fruits, vegetables, whole grains, vegetable protein foods, non-dairy calcium foods, and raw nuts and seeds. Eating a diet based on these dietary guidelines will help get the nutrients you need for optimal health. It's not only the best type of diet for wellness, disease prevention and longevity, it also provides the right balance for building a healthy nervous system.

83

Pure Water: At the foundation of the pyramid is pure water. We recommend drinking pure distilled water as the best type of water for the body. Drink at least 8 – 8 oz glasses of water daily and even more if lifestyle sports, work, etc. requires it. Read Bragg Water Book, page 212.

Whole Grains: Whole grains are the next level of the pyramid. Avoid all process, refined grain products and eat only unrefined, whole grain bread and cereal products. Grains such as whole wheat, brown rice, oats, millet, quinoa, as well as 100% whole grain breads and cereals are the best. One serving of whole grains is equal to 1 slice whole grain bread, 1 ounce ready-to-eat whole grain cereal, 1 cup cooked whole grains such as brown rice, oatmeal or other grains, 1 cup whole wheat (or other whole grain) pasta or noodles, and 1 ounce other whole grain products. We recommend eating 3– 4 servings of whole grains a day.

Vegetables: We recommend eating as many of your vegetables organic and raw (uncooked, in salads, garnishes, juices, etc.) as possible! When you cook vegetables, do not overcook them. Steaming or lightly stir frying is best.

The more colorful your vegetables, the better they are for your health as they contain more valuable nutrients and healthful phytochemicals. Eat a wide variety of vegetables daily. One vegetable serving is equal to 1 cup cooked vegetables or 1 cup raw uncooked vegetables, 1 cup salad, ¾ cup vegetable juice. We recommend having 6 to 8 or more vegetable servings daily.

Fruits: Like vegetables, the more colorful the fruits the better they are for you. Try to have organic fruits as much as possible. One serving of fruit is equal to 1 medium apple, banana, orange, pear or other fruit, ½ cup fruit, ½ cup of fruit juice or ¼ cup dried fruit. We recommend eating 4 to 6 servings or more of organic fruits daily.

Calcium Foods: These are plant-derived calcium-rich foods. Plant source of calcium are healthier than dairy products because they do not contain saturated fats or cholesterol. Health calcium-rich foods contains foods such as soymilk, tofu, broccoli and green leafy vegetables. Examples of serving sizes of plant-derived calcium-rich foods include; 1 cup soymilk, ½ cup tofu, ⅓ cup almonds, 1 cup cooked or 2 cups of high calcium raw greens (kale, collards, broccoli, bok choy or other Chinese greens), 1 cup of calcium-rich beans (e.g. soy, white, navy, Great Northern), ½ cup seaweed, 1 tablespoon blackstrap molasses, 5 or more figs. We recommend having 4 to 6 servings of healthy non-dairy sources of calcium rich foods daily.

Beans and Legumes: This group are the healthy protein foods. Vegetable protein foods are more optimal compared to animal protein foods. Vegetable proteins do not contain the artery clogging saturated fats and cholesterol found in animal foods. They also contain protective factors to prevent heart disease, cancer and diabetes. Vegetable proteins are high quality and provide the body with the essential amino acids that it requires. One serving of vegetable protein foods include; 1 cup cooked legumes (beans, lentils, dried peas), ½ cup firm tofu or tempeh, 1 serving of "veggie meat" alternate (e.g. veggieburger patty or soy patty), 3 tablespoons nut or seed butter, 1 cup soy milk. We recommend having 2 to 3 or more vegetable protein servings daily.

Health Fats, Omega-3 and other Essential Nutrients: This group includes essential and healthy fats and other nutrients. Servings of healthy fats include; 1 teaspoon flax seed oil, 1 tablespoon of Bragg Organic Extra-Virgin olive oil, 3 tablespoons raw walnuts. Other healthy essentials at the top of the pyramid include ground flax seed and nutritional B-Complex supplements that provide vitamin B12, including Bragg Nutritional Yeast (delicious seasoning). Provide your body with the nutritional supplements your body requires for optimal health.

You are Exactly What You Eat and Drink

Of all the various causes of nervous exhaustion and the entire ensemble of conditions that arise with it, incorrect diet probably leads the group. If there is any one thing that must be changed before the body can respond with vigorous health and unlimited Nerve Force, it is the average American diet. To help relieve the strain, stress and tensions that threaten our lives, we must **eat adequate amounts of natural, healthy foods** **to supply the body with the important nutrients for building an active brain in a strong, healthy body.**

The Central Nervous System is made and maintained by the food you eat! How can you build a strong Nervous System and maintain it on hot dogs, washed down with caffeine-filled coffee or colas? How can greasy french fried potatoes supply the nervous system with the valuable nutrients that it needs? It cannot!

As we have devitaminized and demineralized our daily foods we have weakened our Central Nervous System. We are surrounded by an avalanche of chemicals which are poisonous and injurious to our health! Our foods are sprayed with poisonous insecticides. Then the food processors incorporate hundreds of food additives and chemicals which may make their products have longer shelf life, but will ultimately also shorten human life.

There's no substitute for a healthy diet of organic fruits, vegetables, grains and legumes. Vitamin deficiency usually occurs only after many weeks or months of intake below recommended levels. – Complete Guide to Natural Healing

---

Organic natural foods are the greatest source for staying healthy!
– Patricia Bragg, N.D., Ph.D., Pioneer Health Crusader

The awful price we pay for our destruction of the B-Complex vitamins in our "civilized" foods is evident in the confusion, discouragement and desire for suicide – combined with the nervousness and excessive fatigue – so common in our lives and world today. In our opinion the excessive use of tobacco, alcohol, coffee, tea, cola drinks and drugs is directly related to a deficiency in B-Complex vitamins. We have carefully studied the dietary habits of people who use these powerful stimulants and drugs and found in every case that these people are suffering from B-Complex vitamin deficiency.

Millions Suffer Vitamin B-Complex Deficiency

People of every age go about their daily business with their vital energies barely above the point of exhaustion. Watch carefully what they eat and you will find they are not eating foods that help to build Nerve Force.

As is typical of a deficiency, the body signals its need for nutrients with cravings. In the case of B-Complex vitamin deficiency, the body signals its craving for food. Through ignorance, however, people often seek to supply this need with incorrect material by stuffing it with the so-called "quick energy" concoctions that contain refined white sugar; such as candy, chewing gum, cakes, cookies, cola drinks, ice cream, pies and other rich, sugary desserts. These may give an apparent temporary "lift," but this false energy is quickly consumed by the body, leaving the real deficiency even greater than before. So whenever you feel what you interpret as a "craving for sweets" – look to your nerves and reach for the B-Complex vitamin supplements instead of sweets and the sugar bowl!

A B-Complex vitamin deficiency is insidious and difficult to detect. Apparently, the troubles seem to be minor – occasional headaches, some colds and joint and stomach pains, or a clogged bowel which has to be whiplashed with a powerful drug laxative. Ask most people suffering from this deficiency, "How are you feeling today?" Since the trouble seems to be minor, their reply will usually be, *I feel great!* They have had the ailment so long that they have learned to live with it and think nothing of it.

So many people have not the slightest idea what "feeling great" really means! They go on their merry way until Mother Nature finally will not take any more abuses, and then they have a complete nervous breakdown.

Folic Acid Helps Protect the Blood

Folic acid plays a vital role in the smooth functioning of a healthy body. Long revered as a brain food, it's needed for growth of red and white blood cells and the body's energy production. Deficiencies of folic acid, B6 and B12 can lead to serious conditions such as depression, anxiety, insomnia, immune system problems and dangerously high homocysteine levels. Two must-read books by Kilmer S. McCully, M.D. *The Homocysteine Revolution* and *The Heart Revolution (amazon.com)* educate the reader about the deadly toxic effects of high homocysteine levels and the tragic results to the cardiovascular system.

High Homocysteine Levels Can Cause Heart, Alzheimer's, Diabetes and Osteoporosis Problems

High homocysteine levels can damage cells that line the blood vessel walls, setting the stage for future cardiovascular disease and increasing problems with Alzheimer's, diabetes, osteoporosis and kidney diseases. When having a physical, demand a blood panel test that includes your homocysteine level. Dr. McCully says the safest level is 6 to 8 mcm/L, other studies agree.

For every 10% rise in homocysteine levels, there's an equal risk of developing severe coronary disease and osteoporosis. In patients with heart disease, the risk of death 4 to 5 years after diagnosis, was related to the amount of homocysteine in the plasma. Everyone produces this substance naturally, but the homocysteine level can dangerously rise with heavy meat eating and when the body is sluggish (*lack of exercise, fruits, vegetables, water, etc.*), it then fails to convert it to safe, non-damaging amino acids.

In most cases, therapy with various B vitamins and a healthy menu of fresh organic fruits and vegetables offers the B vitamins necessary to reduce high homocysteine levels. But a "normal" American diet doesn't supply enough B vitamins to adequately detoxify homocysteine. This has been scientifically documented by Dr. McCully.

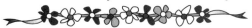

High homocysteine blood level (safe is 6-8 mcm/L) and dietary deficiencies of vitamins (B6, B12, folic acid and CoQ10) are underlying causes of heart, osteoporosis, diabetes and kidney diseases. – Kilmer S. McCully, M.D.
See websites: homocysteine.com, sinatramd.com and www.bu.edu

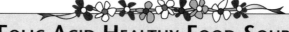

Folic Acid Healthy Food Sources

– The Health Nutrient Bible, Lynn Sonberg

Folic Acid Food Source	MICROGRAMS
Spinach, (raw or steamed) 1 Cup	262
Asparagus, (raw or steamed) 1 Cup	176
Lima Beans, (cooked) 1 Cup	156
Broccoli, (raw or steamed) 1 Cup	108
Wheat Germ, $\frac{1}{4}$ Cup	106
Beets, (raw or steamed) 1 Cup	90
Cauliflower, (raw or steamed) 1 Cup	64
Orange (navel), 1 Cup	47
Cantaloupe, $\frac{1}{2}$ melon	46
Cabbage, (raw or steamed) 1 Cup	40
Tofu, firm $\frac{1}{2}$ Cup	37

B Vitamins & Folic Acid Are Heart Protectors

Dr. Kilmer S. McCully pioneered the Homocysteine Revolution. Here are more positive facts from him: *high homocysteine levels are easily corrected in most people with B-vitamins. B6, B12 and folic acid help reduce homocysteine levels in the blood. This is especially important for those who are at risk for cardiovascular problems, because 1 in every 3 people with cardiovascular disease have dangerously high homocysteine levels (safe level is 6-8 mcm/L).* Godfrey Oakley, M.D., of Centers for Disease Control and Prevention, says *there is strong evidence from over 200 studies that increased intake of folic acid (from foods or supplements) help prevent heart disease.* (Read *Bragg Heart Book*, page 212 for more heart info.)

In addition to supplements, folic acid is found in dates, nutritional yeast, brown rice, mushrooms and more as the list above shows. Folic acid works best taken with vitamin C, B6 and B12, and CoQ10 (see bottom of page 94).

Some doctors prescribe short-term relief to sufferers of angina with nitroglycerin (nitrolingual) spray and digitalis (foxglove) medications. Both increase blood flow to the heart, but in different ways. The former relaxes the veins, increasing blood supply to the heart. The latter makes the heart muscles contract more forcefully (see page 128). It's important to keep in mind that these merely offer temporary relief. The best healthy heart results come from living The Bragg Healthy Lifestyle.

Grapefruit-Seed Extract has a high concentration of antioxidant bioflavonoids.

Foods Rich in the B Vitamin Family

You must plan your meals to be sure that you get all of the B-family vitamins. There are so many delicious foods that will give you this all-important factor in building powerful Nerve Force. Here are some main ones:

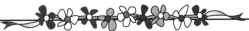

- **Bragg Nutritional Yeast** is rich in B12 and B-Complex vitamins (see page 216) and is our favorite and so delicious. We keep the container on our table for sprinkling over salads, soups, potatoes, casseroles, beans, rice, pasta, veggies, and even delicious over popcorn (page 114). Also remember to use Bragg Liquid Aminos, a nutritious all purpose seasoning (page 214) to add new healthy taste delights to your foods.
- **Nuts, Raw and Unsalted** are best.
- **Whole Grains** such as barley and most 100% whole grain flours – rye, buckwheat flour, corn meal, etc.
- **Beans, dried and raw – Legumes and Lentils** such as lima, soy and green beans as well as fresh and dried, and green peas, etc.
- **Raw Wheat Germ and Rice Bran**
- **Vegetables and Greens** as collards, turnip, kale, spinach mustard greens, broccoli and cabbage.
- **Fruits** such as oranges, grapefruit, bananas, avocados and cantaloupe.
- **Mushrooms** all varieties, fresh and dried.
- **Herbs** alfalfa, cayenne, chamomile, eyebright, fennel, ginseng, parsley, peppermint, sage, rose hips, and more.
- **Molasses** Blackstrap.

89

Bread is called the staff of life, but we shudder at the thought of trying to sustain life on the commercial white breads of today! The best way to be assured of a 100% nutritious loaf of bread – containing all the B-Complex vitamins, vitamin E, Calcium and other nutrients necessary for "the staff of life" – is to bake your own bread.

The following dough recipe can make a variety of breads, rolls, pitas, etc. rich in the B-Complex vitamins. You will have stronger nerves – your payment for the effort it takes to make these natural staff of life taste delights.

Bake Your Own "Live" Healthy Bread
Here's our favorite dough recipe for healthy breads, rolls & pizzas:

2 ¼ cups distilled/purified water
2-3 Tbsps honey, or Stevia (10 drops)
3 teaspoons active dry yeast dissolve
   in warm water 10 minutes

1 cup raw wheat germ
5 cups organic unsifted,
   stone-ground, 100%
   whole wheat flour

Stir raw honey and yeast in 2¼ cups warm distilled water for ten minutes. Add flour and raw wheat germ. Mix well until dough is soft and then knead 5 minutes, then form into 1-2 loaf pans or 2-3 smaller loaves, place in pans brushed with Bragg Organic Olive Oil.

Place on top of stove or in warm oven to let dough rise, leaving oven door open to keep temperature at 80°F. This temperature is often maintained in most ovens by means of the gas pilot alone. If electric, set thermostat to 80°F. Let dough rise (usually hour) to top of baking pan, usually about twice its size. Then gently close oven door and turn heat to 350°F to 375°F. Bake approximately 40 minutes. Watch for when brown crust is formed and bread is drawing slightly from sides of pan, then you know bread is done. Remove from pans, brush lightly with Bragg Organic Olive Oil to keep crust soft and let loaves cool away from drafts. *(Breadmakers are fun and easy to do also.)*

Remember 100% organic whole grains are rich in vital nutrients. **For Variety:** substitute 1-2 cups various grains, organic cornmeal, rice polishings, oatmeal, barley, rye, soy flour, etc. in place of equal amount of whole wheat flour. Try also nutritious, delicious varieties of chopped nuts, sunflower seeds, dates, raisins, figs, prunes, soy cheeses molasses, garlic, herbs, etc. and add to dough mixture.

If you really want to eat a natural, healthy diet you will find time *(try it – it's fun)* and even try a breadmaker to bake your own breads, rolls, pizzas, etc. When people make excuses of being too busy to bake health breads and eat healthy meals, what they are really saying is they are too tired, or weak-willed to make the effort. The sad thing is that they will stay that way until they make the big effort to change and improve their lifestyle!

At mealtime come hither and eat of the bread and dip it in apple cider vinegar and olive oil (as in bible days!). – Ruth 2:14

Take wheat and barley and beans and lentils, and millet and spelt; put them in a single vessel and make bread out of them. – Ezekiel 4:9

Your Nerves Need Plenty of Calcium

We are generally more deficient in calcium than in any of the 30 other minerals the body needs to maintain health and sufficient Nerve Force. Calcium levels in the correct proportion give us sound teeth, strong bones, nerves of steel, good muscle and skin tone, a regular heart beat, an erect posture, a sharp mind and healthy vital organs. If your blood calcium level drops too much you may become nervous, cross, moody, depressed, grouchy and irritated. Calcium helps control your health and moods as it shapes your entire personality.

Calcium is all-important for proper functioning of the nerves. This mineral helps to transport impulses through the nerves from one part of the body to the other. Without calcium, you would not be able to pull your hand away from a hot stove, get out of the way of an oncoming car or even taste the food you eat! Calcium deficiency may cause cramps or convulsions, heart palpitations or a slow pulse. Calcium also helps maintain the body's delicate acid-alkaline balance, Bragg Vinegar helps also.

Calcium deficiencies can be readily recognized by stunted growth, decayed teeth and brittle or porous bones which show up in x-rays. It is more difficult, however, to recognize calcium deficiencies that produce changes in the soft tissues. Yet these are the warning signs which we must learn to detect in order to prevent unnecessary misery and physical handicaps.

Only 1% of the body's calcium is used by the soft tissues. But if this essential 1% is lacking it flashes a danger signal of calcium deficiency. The most noticeable sign is extreme nervousness. Without the proper amount of calcium in the blood, the nerves cannot send messages. Tension and strain result. It is impossible for the body to relax. This is apparent in children who are highly emotional. It shows first in a mean and unpleasant disposition, fretful crying and temper tantrums which can develop into muscular twitching, spasms and even convulsions.

Nutrition directly affects growth, development, reproduction, well-being of an individual's physical and mental condition. Health depends upon nutrition more than on any other single factor. – Dr. William H. Sebrell, Jr.

Calcium Deficiencies Cause Nervous Habits

Both adults and children reveal calcium deficiencies through nervous habits – such as biting the fingernails, continuous restless movements of hands and feet, constant gum chewing, picking at the nose and ears or scratching the head continually. They cannot sit still for any length of time, and there is often an uncontrollable trembling of hands and fingers – especially in adults. People deficient in calcium are usually quite irritable, flying off the handle at the slightest provocation and often going into an emotional tantrum. They may experience spells of uncontrollable weeping and be inclined to wallow in self pity. They are also "jumpy" and become upset or alarmed at the slightest noise. As already noted, calcium deficiency is a major contributing cause to the adverse changes in personality that are the result of low Nerve Force.

Fortunately the opposite is also true. During our long experience in the field of Natural Living, we have seen the meanest, grouchiest, most irritable and nervous people undergo a personality change for the better – a transformation into happy, friendly, self-reliant people – after they change their way of living and following the wonderful and wise Health Laws of Mother Nature.

You too can make some great improvements in your life and personality by obeying the Laws of Mother Nature. Remember that you first have to live with yourself. We know you do not wish to live with an unhappy, restless and irritable person. It is your birthright to be happy and feel fine all the time! But it is strictly an "inside job". It's #1 on the do-it-yourself list. If you are not a well adjusted and happy person, then you should start today to do something about it! Having put in over 95 combined years of research and study on this subject, we believe we can help you to help yourself to build powerful Nerve Force and a happier life.

To help you plan your meals so that you get plenty of calcium in your daily diet, there is a list of the foods that are richest in this important mineral on the next page. Try to get some of these foods into your diet daily.

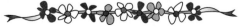

The purpose of life is to live a life of purpose. – Robert Byrne

Calcium Content Chart of Some Common Foods

Calcium Food Source	mgs	Calcium Food Source	mgs
Almonds, 1 oz	80	Kale, (raw/steamed) 1C	180
Artichokes, (steamed) 1C	51	Kohlrabi, (steamed) 1C	40
Beans, (kidney, pinto, red) 1C	89	Mustard Greens, 1C	138
Beans, (great northern, navy) 1C	128	Oatmeal, 1C	120
Beans, (white) 1C	161	Orange, 1 large	96
Blackstrap Molasses, 1 Tbsp	137	Prunes, 4 whole	45
Bok Choy, (steamed) 1C	158	Raisins, 4 oz.	45
Broccoli, (raw/steamed) 1C	178	Rhubarb, (cooked) 1C	105
Brussel Sprouts, (steamed) 1C	56	Rutabaga, (steamed) 1C	72
Buckwheat pancake, 1	99	Sesame Seeds, (unhulled) 1 oz	381
Cabbage, (raw/steamed) 1C	50	Soybeans, 1C	73
Cauliflower, (raw/steamed) 1C	34	Soymilk, fortified	150
Collards, (steamed) 1C	152	Spinach, (raw/steamed) 1C	244
Corn Tortilla	60	Tofu, firm ½ C	258
Cornbread, 1 piece	28	Turnip greens, 1C	198
Figs, (5 medium)	135	Whole Wheat Bread, 1 slice	17

Sources: *Back to Eden,* Jethro Kloss; *Health Nutrient Bible,* Lynne Sonberg; website: www.vrg.org/nutrition/calcium.htm, chart by Brenda Davis, R.D.

93

Benefit From Natural Foods Rich in Calcium

There are some very fine sources of calcium other than milk. Scientists feel that the most bioavailable form of calcium supplement is calcium citrate. We prefer the calcium found in kale, spinach, corn, beans, veggies, soy tofu and sesame seeds. In fact, as Dr. Lynch and Dr. Neal Barnard point out, all natural foods contain appreciable amounts of calcium. This chart above shows foods that contain large amounts of calcium you should include in your diet.

Read 2 important books on milk & why best to avoid milk:

- *Mad Cows and Milk Gate* by Virgil Hulse, M.D.
- *Milk, the Deadly Poison* by Robert Cohen

Both books on *amazon.com*. Also visit these websites:
- *www.notmilk.com* • *www.strongbones.org*
- *pcrm.org* (Physicians Committee for Responsible Medicine)

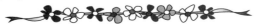

Many osteoporosis studies consistently conclude that vegetarians have stronger bones than meat-eaters. Many world-wide studies show that it's healthier to avoid meat and dairy products for optimum heart health.

It's strange that some men will drink and eat anything put before them, but will check very carefully the oil they put in their car.

Milk is Not a Good Source of Calcium

Nearly everyone has the idea that the problem of calcium deficiency will be solved if they just drink milk. This is not completely true. In the first place, practically all the milk in U.S. is pasteurized, which robs and greatly reduces the availability of milk's calcium (see page 93 and web: *www.notmilk.com*).

Dr. Harold D. Lynch – famous author, researcher and physician – said recently *almost fanatic use of milk as a beverage has added more complications than benefits to child nutrition.* He further states *milk may often be a primary cause of poor nutrition in children!*

This might be due to the fact that proportionate amounts of Vitamins A and D and phosphorus must be present in the metabolism for the proper absorption and utilization of calcium by the body; another reason why proper nutrition and a balanced diet are so important!

Whole milk is a carrier of large amounts of saturated fat (cholesterol) and can lead to atherosclerosis. This food is just for cow's babies. It's wise for humans if they wish to maintain a healthy heart for a long life to eliminate milk!

Calcium Can Help Tame PMS

The mental and physical complaints associated with premenstrual syndrome (PMS) which some women endure monthly prior to menstruation, can be reduced greatly by supplementing with calcium, according to several studies. James G. Penland, Ph.D., a psychologist for U.S. Dept. of Agriculture, placed a group of women with PMS symptoms on a food diet containing 600 mg of calcium. He then gave half the group 700 mg more of calcium in supplement form, and the other half a placebo (sugar pill). Women taking calcium supplement reported 70% less pain, such as backaches and cramping, and 80% less water retention. **On the emotional side, 90% of women taking the supplement experienced less crying, irritability and depression.** Once again, calcium lived up to its name as "the miracle mineral." A multi-mineral with calcium, magnesium, etc. and CoQ10 and 3 mgs of boron is best.

Nature, time and patience are the three greatest physicians. – Irish Proverb

Locations in the Body Where Osteoporosis, Arthritis, Pain and Misery Hit the Hardest

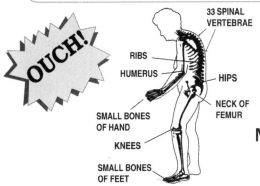

OUCH!

33 SPINAL VERTEBRAE
RIBS
HUMERUS
SMALL BONES OF HAND
KNEES
SMALL BONES OF FEET
HIPS
NECK OF FEMUR

OSTEOPOROSIS
Affects over 30 Million and Kills 400,000 Americans Annually

Boron
Miracle Trace Mineral For Healthy Bones

BORON – A trace mineral for healthier bones that also helps the body absorb more vital calcium, minerals and necessary hormones! Good sources are most organic veggies, fresh and sun-dried fruits, prunes, raw nuts and soybeans.

The U.S. Department of Agriculture's Human Nutrition Lab in Grand Forks, North Dakota, says boron is usually found in soil and in foods, but many Americans eat a diet low in boron. They conducted a 17 week study which showed a daily 3 to 6 mgs boron supplement enabled participants to reduce loss (demineralization) of calcium, phosphorus and magnesium from their bodies. This loss is usually caused by eating processed fast foods and lots of meat, salt, sugar and fat and a dietary lack of fresh vegetables, fruits and whole grains. (*all-natural.com*)

95

After 8 weeks on boron, participants' calcium loss was cut 40%. It also helped double important hormone levels vital in maintaining calcium and healthy bones. Millions on estrogen replacement therapy for osteoporosis* may want to use boron as a healthier choice.* Also consider natural progesterone (2%) raw yam cream. For pain and joint healing use Braggzyme (pg. 218), and glucosamine/chondroitin/MSM combo (caps or liquid).

Scientific studies show women benefit from healthy lifestyle that includes gentle vitamin D3 sunshine and exercise (even weight lifting) to maintain healthier bones, combined with a low-fat, high-fiber, carbohydrate, and fresh organic fruits, salads, sprouts, greens and vegetable diet. This lifestyle helps protect against heart disease, high blood pressure, cancer and many other ailments. I'm happy to see science now agrees with my Dad who first stated these health truths in 1920's.

**For more hormone and osteoporosis facts read pioneer John Lee, M.D.'s book*
– What Your Doctor May Not Tell You About Menopause. (amazon.com)

Macafem, a non-estrogenic herb, stimulates hormonal glands to produce the necessary hormones naturally to help menopausal symptoms. – Macafem.com

- Bone and muscle aches and pains, especially lower back.

- The body feels heavy, tired and it's an effort to move.

- Shooting pains when straightening up after leaning over.

- Dizziness upon straightening up after leaning over.

- Morning dull headaches upon arising and when stressed.

- Dull, faded-looking hair that lacks sheen and luster.

- The scalp is itchy and dry. Dandruff, premature hair thinning or balding may occur.

- The hair is unmanageable, mats, often looks straw-like, and is sometimes extremely dry and other times oily.

- The eyes itch, feel sore and uncomfortable and appear bloodshot and watery. Also, eyelids may be granulated with white matter collecting in the corners.

- The eyes tire easily and will not focus as they should.

- You tire physically and mentally with the slightest effort.

- Loss of mental alertness and onset of confusion, making decisions difficult. The memory fails, making you forget familiar names and places you should easily remember.

- You become easily irritable and impatient with family, friends and loved ones and even with your business and social acquaintances.

- You feel nervous, depressed, in a mental fog, and have difficulty getting things done due to mental and muscle fatigue. Even the slightest effort can leave you exhausted, upset and trembling.

- At times, your hands and feet get chilled, even in warm weather, which is a sign of potassium deficiency.

96

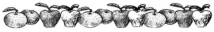

Hippocrates, the Father of Medicine, in 400 B.C., treated his patients with amazing raw Apple Cider Vinegar because he recognized its powerful cleansing and healing qualities. It is a naturally occurring antibiotic and antiseptic that fights the germs and bacteria in the body.

Potassium is the key mineral in the constellation of minerals; it's so important to every living thing that without it there would be no life. Bragg Organic Raw Apple Cider Vinegar is a natural potassium source.

Nature's Miracle Phytonutrients Help Prevent Cancer:

Make sure to get your daily dose of these naturally occurring, cancer-fighting super foods – phytonutrients that are abundant in apples, tomatoes, onions, garlic, beans, legumes, soybeans, cabbage, cauliflower, broccoli, citrus fruits, etc. The champions with the highest count of phytonutrients go to apples and tomatoes.

Class	Food Sources	Action
PHYTOESTROGEN ISOFLAVONES	Soy products, flaxseed, seeds & nuts, yams, alfalfa & red clover sprouts, licorice root (not candy)	Helps block some cancers, & aids in menopausal symptoms and helps improve the memory
PHYTOSTEROLS	Plant oils, corn, soy, sesame, safflower, wheat, pumpkin	Blocks hormonal role in cancers, inhibits uptake of cholesterol from diet
SAPONINS	Yams, beets, beans, cabbage, nuts, soybeans	Helps prevent cancer cells from multiplying
TERPENES	Carrots, winter squash, sweet potatoes, yams, apples, cantaloupes	Antioxidants – protects DNA from free radical-induced damage
	Tomatoes & its sauces, tomato-based products	Helps block UVA & UVB and offers help to protect against cancers, prostate, etc.
	Spinach, kale, beets & turnip greens, cabbage	Protects eyes from macular degeneration
	Red chile peppers	Keeps carcinogens from binding to DNA
QUERCETIN (& FLAVONOIDS)	Apples, especially the skins, red onions and only green tea without caffeine	Strong cancer fighter, protects heart & arteries. Reduces pain, allergy & asthma symptoms
	Citrus fruits (flavonoids)	Promotes protective enzymes
PHENOLS	Apples, fennel, parsley, carrots, alfalfa, cabbage	Helps prevent blood clotting & has some anticancer properties
	Cinnamon	Promotes healthy blood sugar and glucose metabolism
	Citrus fruits, broccoli, cabbage, cucumbers, green peppers, tomatoes	Antioxidants – flavonoids, block membrane receptor sites for certain hormones
	Apples, grape seeds	Strong antioxidants; fights germs & bacteria, strengthens immune system, veins & capillaries
	Grapes, especially skins	Antioxidant, antimutagen; promotes detoxification. Acts as carcinogen inhibitors
	Yellow & green squash	Antihepatotoxic, antitumor
SULFUR COMPOUNDS	Onions & garlic, (fresh is always best) Red onions (our favorite) also contain Quercetin. Onions help keep doctor away.	Promotes liver enzymes, inhibits cholesterol synthesis, reduces triglycerides, lowers blood pressure, improves immune response, fights infections, germs & parasites

Food and Product Summary

Today, many American foods are highly processed or refined, robbing them of essential nutrients, vitamins, minerals and enzymes. Many also contain harmful, toxic and dangerous chemicals. The research findings and experience of top nutritionists, physicians and dentists have led to the discovery that devitalized foods are a major cause of poor health, illness, cancer and premature death. The enormous increase in the last 70 years of degenerative diseases such as heart disease, diabetes, arthritis and dental decay verify this belief. Scientific research has shown that most of these afflictions can be prevented and that others, once established, can be arrested or even reversed through nutritional and healthy lifestyle methods.

Enjoy Super Health with Natural Foods

1. **RAW FOODS:** Fresh fruits and raw vegetables organically grown are always best. Enjoy nutritious variety garden salads with raw vegetables, sprouts, raw nuts and seeds.
2. **VEGETABLES and PROTEINS:**
   a. Legumes, lentils, brown rice, soybeans, and all beans.
   b. Nuts and seeds, raw and unsalted (lightly roasted okay).
   c. We prefer healthier vegetarian proteins. If you must have animal protein, then be sure it's hormone–free, and organically fed and no more than 1 or 2 times a week.
   d. Dairy products – fertile range-free eggs (*not over 3-4 weekly*), unprocessed hard cheese and feta goat's cheese. We choose not to use dairy products. Try the healthier non-dairy soy, rice, nut, and almond milks and soy cheeses, delicious soy yogurt and soy and rice ice cream.
3. **FRUITS and VEGETABLES:** Organically grown is always best, grown without use of poisonous sprays and toxic chemical fertilizers. Urge markets to stock organic produce! Steam, bake, sauté and wok vegetables as short a time as possible to retain best nutritional content, flavor and use raw veggies in salads, sandwiches, etc. Also enjoy fresh juices.
4. **100% WHOLE GRAIN CEREALS, BREADS and FLOURS:** They contain important B-Complex vitamins, vitamin E, minerals, fiber and the important unsaturated fatty acids.
5. **COLD or EXPELLER-PRESSED VEGETABLE OILS:** Bragg Organic Extra Virgin Olive Oil (is best), soy, sunflower, flax and sesame oils are excellent sources of healthy, essential, unsaturated fatty acids. We still use oils sparingly.

Enjoy Lighter, Smaller Vegetarian Dinners

It seems to be an American custom for people to eat their biggest meal in the evening. From a standpoint of heart attacks, this is the worst time to eat a big meal . . . especially a meal with a preponderance of fat. It has been definitively established by researchers that the blood is more likely to clot 2 to 8 hours following a meal with a high fat intake. It would therefore seem logical to avoid heavy meals – particularly in the evening – to minimize the chances of intravascular clotting. The occurrence of a heart attack after eating a heavy meal has been recognized by doctors for years. Just think of how often you read or hear about a man in his prime dying of a heart attack while in bed at night.

Retired people can regulate their mealtimes easily. Also working people can dine at an earlier hour in the evening and can certainly regulate their diet to promote health and longevity and prolong their golden years!

Light, healthy vegetarian meal is ideal for early evening

It can begin with raw combination salad (see page 115) with Bragg Vinaigrette or Ginger Dressing. Follow with 2-3 lightly cooked vegetables – green beans, zucchini, peas, corn, carrots, kale, okra, vegetable stir-fry, etc. Several nights a week add a baked potato – but do not drench this potato in fat! Season it with spray of Bragg Aminos, Bragg Kelp or Sprinkle (24 herbs & spices) and Bragg Organic Extra Virgin Olive Oil instead of butter.

Now we are not telling you that the price you must pay to avoid a heart attack and live a longer life is to give up good flavor. Not at all! As mentioned previously, French dishes, soups, salads, potatoes and vegetables, etc. are world famous and among the best heart-healthy recipes. A good French chef rarely uses salt and cooks with very little fat. The secrets of French flavor lie in the use of herbs, garlic, olive oil, onions, green peppers and mushrooms.

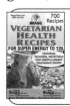

The Bragg Vegetarian Health Recipe Book
Over 700 Delicious, Nutritious Recipes
For Super Energy and Long Life to 120!
See back pages 211-213 for booklist.

Instead of medicine, fast for a day. – Plutarch, Greek Philosopher, 83 A.D.

7 Ways to Keep Blood Sugar Levels Low

Australian researcher Dr. Jennie Brand-Miller cites in her new book *The Glucose Revolution* (*amazon.com*), that when you eat a carbohydrate – any sugary or starchy food – your blood sugar goes up. If it rises slowly, that's ideal; however, if it soars quickly, this could lead to serious health threats. Researchers at Harvard Medical School have also cited that a spike in blood sugar can double or triple your risk of developing Type 2 (adult onset) diabetes.

Dr. Brand-Miller has created a Glycemic Index (GI) that ranks foods based on how quickly they raise blood sugar. High-glycemic-index foods make blood sugar jump quickly; Low-glycemic-index foods cause a slower rise.

● Eat health giving legumes with abandon, such as lentils, soybeans, lima and kidney beans, etc., for they promote a gradual blood sugar rise and have a low-glycemic-index.

● Don't worry about carrots spiking blood sugar. Wide reports that carrots are bad for blood sugar are wrong.

● Add Bragg Apple Cider Vinegar or Bragg Salad Dressings over foods. Studies show only a few tsps of salad dressing, over veggies, etc. helps lower blood sugar because the acid slows stomach emptying and promotes better digestion.

● Eating organic brown rice, lentils and whole grain pastas are healthy and filling. They help normalize blood sugar and reduce appetite that helps in weight loss.

● If you snack, choose fresh organic fruits, even popcorn.

● Eat fresh, organic vegetables. Think of salad vegetables as "free" foods, with no significant impact on blood sugar or weight. It's best to avoid fatty foods, sugars, meat, etc.

● Avoid all processed, refined foods: refined breads, cereals, cookies, crackers, desserts etc. These refined starches zip through your digestive tract, raising your blood sugar.

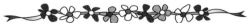

Less Sodium and Sugar in Processed Foods: *New 2011 U.S. Government nutrition guidelines urging Americans to use less sodium and sugar in their diets places pressure on the food industry to reformulate process foods. Walmart recently announced a 5-year plan to reformulate its store-brand packaged foods and drop its prices on fruits and vegetables. Kraft Foods, has vowed to reduce sodium by an average of 10% by 2012, and plans to reformulate more than 1,000 products. Campbell Soup has replaced regular salt with smaller amounts of sea salt in some of their products.*

Avoid These Processed, Refined, Harmful Foods

Once you realize the harm caused to your body by unhealthy refined, chemicalized, deficient foods, you'll want to eliminate these "killer" foods. Also avoid microwaved foods! Follow The Bragg Healthy Lifestyle to provide the basic, healthy nourishment to maintain your health.

- Refined sugar, artificial sweeteners (toxic aspartame) or their products such as jams, jellies, preserves, marmalades, yogurts, ice cream, sherbets, Jello, cake, candy, cookies, all chewing gum, colas & diet drinks, pies, pastries, & all sugared fruit juices & fruits canned in sugar syrup. **(Health Stores have delicious healthy replacements, such as Stevia, raw honey, 100% maple syrup, & agave nectar, so seek & buy the best.)**

- White flour products such as white bread, wheat-white bread, enriched flours, rye bread that has white flour in it, dumplings, biscuits, buns, gravy, pasta, pancakes, waffles, soda crackers, pizza, ravioli, pies, pastries, cakes, cookies, prepared & commercial puddings & ready-mix bakery products. Most are made with dangerous (oxy-cholesterol) powdered milk & powdered eggs. **(Health Stores have huge variety of 100% whole grain organic products, delicious breads, crackers, pastas, desserts, etc.)**

- Salted foods, such as corn chips, potato chips, pretzels, crackers & nuts.

- Refined white rices & pearled barley. • Fried fast foods. • Indian ghee.

- Refined, sugared (also aspartame) dry processed cereals – cornflakes, etc.

- Foods that contain Olestra, palm & cottonseed oil. These oils are not fit for human consumption & should be totally avoided.

- Peanuts & peanut butter that contain hydrogenated, hardened oils & any peanuts with mold & all molds that can cause allergies.

- Margarine – combines heart-deadly trans-fatty acids and saturated fats.

- Saturated fats & hydrogenated oils – enemies that clog the arteries.

- Coffee – even decaffeinated, caffeinated (even if in green) teas & alcohol. Also all caffeinated and sugared water-juices, all cola and soft drinks.

- Fresh pork and products. • Fried, fatty, greasy meats. • Irradiated GMO foods.

- Smoked meats, such as ham, bacon, sausage & smoked fish.

- Luncheon meats, hot dogs, salami, bologna, corned beef, pastrami & packaged meats containing dangerous sodium nitrate or nitrite.

- Dried fruits containing sulphur dioxide – a toxic preservative.

- Don't eat chickens or turkeys that have been injected with hormones or fed with commercial poultry feed containing any drugs or toxins.

- Canned soups - read labels for sugar, salt, starch, flour & preservatives.

- Foods containing benzoate of soda, salt, sugar, cream of tartar & any additives, drugs, preservatives; irradiated & genetically engineered foods.

- Day-old cooked vegetables, potatoes & pre-mixed, wilted lifeless salads.

- All commercial vinegars: pasteurized, filtered, distilled, white, malt & synthetic vinegars are dead vinegars! (*We use only our Bragg Organic Raw, unfiltered Apple Cider Vinegar with the "Mother Enzyme" as used in olden times.*)

101

Increase Your Stamina and Go Power

If you eat right you will be able to go the distance, whether it's competing in a triathlon or the next marathon work day. It is important to boost stamina by taking advantage of the way energy is released in the body and trying to keep this process from getting bogged down. The body breaks food down into blood sugar, or glucose, which powers the cells. Nutrients such as B vitamins, iron, magnesium and zinc play vital roles in driving this energy-providing process. It's crucial to stamina that you get enough of them. Overindulging in nutrient-rich food can be counterproductive, if the body expends too much energy digesting food that's not immediately needed, then precious energy is wasted.

Stamina – Boosting Foods and Nutrients

- Kidney Beans and Lentils • Water – purified, distilled
- Whole Grain Pastas, Brown Rice, Bran and Cereal
- Spinach, Swiss Chard, and other Leafy Greens

Vitamins and minerals, which play important roles in all of the chemical processes of the body, help maintain stamina in two primary ways: helping your body break down the high-energy foods you eat and use as energy; and helping your brain produce chemicals that make you feel energetic for a sustained period. A few of the most important nutrients when it comes to stamina are: iron, 18-30 mgs. daily; calcium, 250-800 mgs. daily; and magnesium, 125-400 mgs. daily. (See page 128.)

The Stamina Balance

Nutritionists recommend that you get 55 to 60% of your calories from complex carbohydrates like whole-grain bread, cereal, rice, grains and pasta. These provide a slow, steady release of energy and also contain the vitamins and minerals you need to produce energy. Athletes take advantage of this time-released energizing power by "carbo-loading". Balancing carbs with protein-rich foods like beans works well for the normal person.

No man can violate Mother Nature's Laws and escape her penalties.

Boost Your Memory

The mental function of memory allows us to recall ideas, facts, sensations and impressions. There are three types of memory: sensory, short-term and long-term. We never really give memory much thought until we forget where we parked the car or forget an appointment or have trouble remembering a name. There are many factors which affect the memory, such as your overall health, diet, age, hormone levels and some medications. However there are several things you can do to preserve or improve your memory. Scientists are discovering nutrients found in certain foods help enhance the memory and they are easy to include in your meals.

The Brain – Memory Boosting Diet

Consuming a low-fat diet to keep cholesterol in check is the very first step you should take toward improving your memory. This is vital because high cholesterol levels inhibit the flow of oxygen to your brain and cause the memory to falter. The next step is simply to add foods to your diet that benefit brain and nerve function. One serving of grains, soy, brown rice or lentils and five servings of fruits and vegetables provide the nutrients needed to bolster your memory. Certain lifestyle changes that enhance memory are to avoid second-hand smoke and NEVER smoke, or use recreational drugs or alcohol!

Nutrients and Herbs to the Rescue

Ginkgo biloba, ginseng, and rosemary have been used for thousands of years to enhance memory. Studies show that these herbs have antioxidant properties that aid blood and oxygen flow to the brain. Ginkgo also helps boost metabolism and electrical brain activity. Rosemary, known as "the remembrance herb," helps prevent the breakdown of acetylcholine, a brain chemical crucial to memory. Also try Niacin (B3 – 100mg) daily with meal.

Soy products, whole grains and fish oils help boost memory. Lecithin (found in soy beans), wheat germ, Bragg Nutritional Yeast and phytoestrogens in yams, flaxseeds, raw nuts and seeds also help improve memory (page 97).

Cross-Train Your Brain: *keep it youthful – brain exchange with family, friends, chat groups & learn new challenges, games, sports, dancing, gardening, etc.*

Soybean Products for Healthy Nerves

We have been recommending the use of soybeans and its products to the health-conscious people of America since 1912. Lecithin – of which the soybean is the richest source – is not just important in the digestion of fats. The functioning of the nervous system and the glands are greatly aided by the phospholipids, one of the most important constituents of lecithin. That's why it's found in the nervous system and in every cell of the body. Nutritional Science teaches us that the nerves and cardiovascular system both require lecithin and the vitamin B-complex rich foods, see pages 86-89.

Bragg Introduces Miracles of Soybeans

Over 88 years ago my father introduced Bragg Liquid Aminos to the health-minded as a way to help them increase natural, life-building vegetable protein intake in a form that's easily digestible and delicious to use! It's a liquid form of soy protein from pure, healthy (certified non-genetically engineered) soybeans – a 100% health product that contains no coloring agents, preservatives or added sodium. Lack of adequate Amino Acids in your body may make it impossible for the vitamins and minerals to perform their specific duties. Amino Acids are inseparably interwoven with vitamins and minerals for good sound nutrition. Bragg Liquid Aminos contains no meat, and adds delicious natural flavors and zest to most all foods by sprinkling or spraying on foods. It's the most delicious, nutritious and unique gourmet health seasoning, for it contains 16 important vital Amino Acids and Isoflavones for super health.

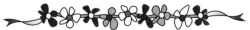

*There is a high concentration of lecithin in the sheathing around the brain, spinal cord and nerves. Lecithin comes in granules, liquid and capsules from the diversified, healthy soybean. **Lecithin is a natural fat emulsifier** and increases vital choline levels. Choline is important to the central nervous system and helps reduce anxiety.*

WHAT ARE AMINO ACIDS? *They're the building blocks of proteins and all our organs and tissues. They are essential for production of energy within ourselves, for detoxification and for the vital transmission of nerve impulses. In short, they are the very soup of life, and are almost always overlooked and neglected.* – H.J. Hoegerman, M.D., (Bragg Aminos Fan)

Vegetarian Protein % Chart

LEGUMES	%
Soybean Sprouts	54
Soybean Curd (tofu)	43
Soy flour	35
Soybeans	35
Broad Beans	32
Lentils	29
Split Peas	28
Kidney Beans	26
Navy Beans	26
Lima Beans	26
Garbanzo Beans	23

VEGETABLES	%
Spirulina *(Plant Algae)*	60
Spinach	49
New Zealand Spinach	47
Watercress	46
Kale	45
Broccoli	45
Brussels Sprouts	44
Turnip Greens	43
Collards	43
Cauliflower	40
Mustard Greens	39
Mushrooms	38
Chinese Cabbage	34
Parsley	34
Lettuce	34
Green Peas	30
Zucchini	28
Green Beans	26
Cucumbers	24
Dandelion Greens	24
Green Pepper	22
Artichokes	22
Cabbage	22
Celery	21
Eggplant	21
Tomatoes	18
Onions	16
Beets	15
Pumpkin	12
Potatoes	11
Yams	8
Sweet Potatoes	6

GRAINS	%
Wheat Germ	31
Rye	20
Wheat, hard red	17
Wild rice	16
Buckwheat	15
Oatmeal	15
Millet	12
Barley	11
Brown Rice	8

FRUITS	%
Lemons	16
Honeydew Melon	10
Cantaloupe	9
Strawberry	8
Orange	8
Blackberry	8
Cherry	8
Apricot	8
Grape	8
Watermelon	8
Tangerine	7
Papaya	6
Peach	6
Pear	5
Banana	5
Grapefruit	5
Pineapple	3
Apple	1

105

NUTS AND SEEDS	%
Pumpkin Seeds	21
Sunflower Seeds	17
Peanuts	16
Walnuts, black	13
Sesame Seeds	13
Almonds	12
Cashews	12
Macadamia Nuts	9

Data from Nutritive Value of American Foods in Common Units, USDA Agriculture Handbook No. 456. Reprinted with author's permission, from *Diet for a New America* John Robbins (Walpole, NH: Stillpoint Publishing)

Vegetable and Fruit Juices Contain Mother Nature's Distilled Water

No new water has been put on the face of Mother Earth since it was originally formed. Just as the same energy is formed and re-formed, so the same water is used and re-used over and over again by the miracle of Mother Nature. Waters of the earth are purified by distillation. The sun evaporates the water which is collected into clouds. When the clouds become full we have rain and dew – pure, perfectly clean, distilled water, free of all harmful inorganic substances, until polluted!

Years ago, when the late Douglas Fairbanks, Senior, and Dad were close friends, they roamed the South Sea Islands for several months. During that trip Dad came upon an island inhabited by *beautiful, healthy Polynesians* who drank only distilled rain water because the island was surrounded by the Pacific Ocean. Their island was based on porous coral which could not hold water – so they would *only drink rain water* or the fresh, clear, clean water of the green coconut. (Rain water is stored worldwide by millions.) Dad had never seen any finer specimens of humanity than these native South Sea Islanders. There were several doctors on the yacht who thoroughly examined the most mature people on these islands. One heart doctor stated that he had never in his life examined such healthy, well-preserved people.

You may have noted we said only the most mature people were examined by the doctors. *They were so completely unaware of age* that no such word existed in their language! They never celebrated birthdays, so they were forever young – gloriously ageless, not only in years but in body. These older men performed as well in the vigorous native dances as the younger men. They were all beautiful human specimens because they lived their lengthy lives drinking only pure distilled water, eating natural foods and enjoying a happy, healthy lifestyle.

I now live on legumes, vegetables and fruits. No dairy, no meat of any kind, no chicken, no turkey, and very little fish, only once in a while. It changed my metabolism and I lost 24 pounds. I did research and found 82% of people who go on a plant-based diet begin to heal themselves, as I did.
– Bill Clinton, United States President, 1993-2001

The 70% Watery Human

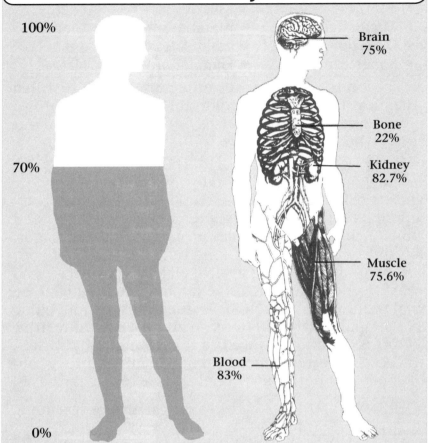

100%

70%

0%

Brain
75%

Bone
22%

Kidney
82.7%

Muscle
75.6%

Blood
83%

107

The amount of water in the human body, averaging 70%, varies considerably and even from one part of the body to another area (illustration on right). A lean man may hold 70% of his weight in body water, while a woman – because of her larger proportion of water-poor fatty tissues – may be only 52% water. The lowering of the water content in the blood is what triggers the hypothalamus, the brain's vital thirst center, to send out its familiar urgent demand for a drink of water! Please obey and drink ample amounts (8 glasses) of purified water daily. *By the time you feel thirsty, you're already dehydrated. – American Running & Fitness Association*

Water Percentage in Various Body Parts:

Teeth	10%	Spleen	75.5%
Bones	22%	Lungs	80%
Cartilage	55%	Blood	83%
Red blood corpuscles	68.7%	Bile	86%
Liver	71.5%	Plasma	90%
Muscle tissue	75%	Lymph	94%
Brain	75%	Saliva	95.5%

Chart shows why 8-10 glasses distilled water daily is important.

Your body suffers when you're water dehydrated. The body's cells are like sponges. It takes time for cells to become hydrated. Daily drink 8 glasses of distilled water.

Water is the Key to All Body Functions!

- Heart
- Circulation
- Digestion
- Bones & Joints
- Muscles
- Metabolism
- Assimilation
- Elimination
- Energy
- Glands
- Sex
- Nerves

The body is 70% water and pure, steam-distilled (chemical-free) water is important for total health. You should drink at least 8 glasses of water daily. Read our book, *Water – The Shocking Truth*, for more info on the importance of pure water. See back pages for booklist.

Pure, distilled water is vitally important in following The Bragg Healthy Lifestyle. Water is the key to all body functions including: digestion, circulation, bones and joints, assimilation, elimination, muscles, nerves, glands, sex and senses. The right kind of water is one of your best natural protections against all kinds of diseases and viral infections, such as influenza and pneumonia. It is a vital factor in all body fluids, tissues, cells, lymph, blood and all glandular secretions. Water holds all nutritive factors in solution, as well as toxins and body wastes, and acts as the main transportation medium throughout the body, for both nutritional and cleansing purposes!

108

Distilled water is the world's purest and best water!

It's excellent for detoxification, fasting and cleansing of cells, organs and body fluids, because it helps carry away harmful toxins, substances, etc. (purified and reverse osmosis water is acceptable also). Water from all chemically treated public water systems – and even from many wells and springs – is likely to be loaded with poisonous chemicals and toxic trace elements. Depending upon the kinds of pipes used in the buildings, the water is likely to be overloaded with lead (from older, soldered pipe joints), zinc (from old-fashioned galvanized pipes) or with copper and cadmium (from copper pipes). These trace elements are released in dangerous quantities by the chemical action of the water flowing against the metals of the pipes.

Distilled water plays vital part in treatment of illness, arthritis, etc. – Dr. Banik

There is only one water that is clean and that is steam distilled water. No other substance on our planet does so much to keep us healthy and get us well as this water does. – Dr. James Balch, Dietary Wellness

Almost every known food may cause some allergic reaction at times. Thus, foods used in elimination diets may cause allergic reactions in some individuals. Some are listed among the Most Common Food Allergies (see below). Since reaction to these foods is generally low, they are widely used in making test diets. By keeping a food journal and tracking your pulse rate after meals you will soon know your problem foods. Allergic foods cause pulse to go up. (Take base pulse before meals and then 30 minutes after meals. If it increases 8-10 beats per minute – check foods for allergies.) See web: *wrc.net/wrcnet_content/dietplans/cocoa_pulse_test.htm*

If your body has a reaction after eating a particular food, especially if it happens each time you eat that food, you may have an allergy. Some allergic reactions are: wheezing, sneezing, stuffy nose, nasal drip or mucus, dark circles, eye watering or waterbags under eyes, headaches, feeling light-headed or dizzy, fast heart beat, stomach or chest pains, diarrhea, extreme thirst, breaking out in a rash, swelling of extremities or stomach bloating, etc. (Read famous Dr. Arthur Coca's book, *The Pulse Test* – available on: *amazon.com*)

If you know what you're allergic to, you're lucky; if you don't, you better find out as fast as possible and eliminate all irritating foods from your diet. To reevaluate your daily life and have a health guide to your future, start a daily journal (8 $^1/_2$ x 11 notebook- enlarge and copy form on next page) of foods eaten, your pulse rate after meals and your reactions, moods, energy levels, weight, elimination and sleep patterns. You will discover the foods and situations causing problems. By charting your diet you will be amazed at the effects of eating certain foods. Dad kept a daily journal for over 70 years.

109

If you are hypersensitive to certain foods, you must omit them from your diet! There are hundreds of allergies and of course it's impossible here to take up each one. Many have allergies to milk, wheat, or some are allergic to all grains. Visit web: *foodallergy.org*. Your daily journal will help you discover and accurately pinpoint the foods and situations causing you problems. Start your journal today!

Most Common Food Allergies

- **MILK:** Butter, Cheese, Cottage Cheese, Ice Cream, Milk, Yogurt, etc.
- **CEREALS & GRAINS:** Wheat, Corn, Buckwheat, Oats, Rye
- **EGGS:** Cakes, Custards, Dressings, Mayonnaise, Noodles
- **FISH:** Shellfish, Crabs, Lobster, Shrimp, Shad Roe
- **MEATS:** Bacon, Beef, Chicken, Pork, Sausage, Veal, Smoked Products
- **FRUITS:** Citrus Fruits, Melons, Strawberries
- **NUTS:** Peanuts, Pecans, Walnuts, chemically dried preserved nuts
- **MISCELLANEOUS:** Chocolate, Cocoa, Coffee, Black & Green (caffeine) Teas, Palm & Cottonseed Oils, MSG & Salt. Allergic reactions often caused by toxic pesticides, sprays, etc. on salad greens, vegetables & fruits, etc.

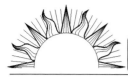

MY DAILY HEALTH JOURNAL

Today is:____/____/____

> ### *I have said my morning resolve and am ready to practice*
> ### *The Bragg Healthy Lifestyle today and every day.*

Yesterday I went to bed at: Today I arose at: Weight:

Today I practiced the No-Heavy Breakfast or No-Breakfast Plan: ☐ yes ☐ no

- For Breakfast I drank: Time:

  For Breakfast I ate: Time:

  Supplements:

- For Lunch I ate: Time:

  Supplements:

- For Dinner I ate: Time:

  Supplements:

- _____Glasses of Water I Drank during the Day

  List Snacks – Kind and When:

- I took part in these physical (walking, gym, etc.) activities today:

Grade each on scale of 1 to 10 (desired optimum health is 10).
- I rate my day for the following categories:

Previous Night's Sleep:	Stress/Anxiety:
Energy Level:	Elimination:
Physical Activity, Exercise:	Health:
Peacefulness:	Accomplishments:
Happiness:	Self-Esteem:

- General Comments, Reactions and To Do List:

Dr. Charles Attwood – Great Health Crusader

As a doctor, humanitarian, strong dedicated health crusader and a devoted pediatrician for over 40 years, and Fellow of the American Academy of Pediatrics, Dr. Charles Raymond Attwood fought many battles against mainstream medicine and big business to ensure the health of people everywhere, particularly children. He championed a low-fat vegetarian menu for children, was a strong health and nutrition activist and an associate of Dr. Benjamin Spock. One major battle occurred in 1996. As a member of the Center for Science in the Public Interest, Dr. Attwood led opposition to the giant Gerber Baby Food Company's practice of diluting its baby foods with water, sugar and starch. He won! Gerber stopped this 40 year crime against America's children. Now their foods are 100% fruits and vegetables. Other baby food companies then followed. See web: *vegsource.com*.

Dr. Attwood held high the banner advocating a low-fat, plant-based diet as the most healthy for youngsters. His highly praised 1995 book, *Low-fat Prescription for Kids* (available *amazon.com*) makes a strong scientific argument for this diet. His research shows to avoid the leading causes of premature death later as adults: heart disease, stroke, cancers, diabetes, etc. it's important children follow his program.

Dr. Attwood's Tips for Low-Fat Shopping

- Spend most of your time in the produce department.
- Try new varieties of produce. Look at those with the most intense colors and remember organic is best!
- Don't forget about pasta made from whole-grains.
- Go straight for the whole-grain breads section.
- Buy unrefined, low-fat, sugarless, high-fiber cereals.
- When buying packaged, canned, frozen foods, read labels.
- Don't underestimate beans – whether dried, frozen or canned, they are delicious and healthy for you.
- Buy low- or no-fat healthy snacks – there's many choices. Careful, some are high in salt, sugar and calories.
- Replace milk and low-fat dairy products with soy, nut and rice milks, and soy and tofu cheeses, etc.

Seek and choose whole foods, organic fruits, vegetables and organic whole grain cereals, breads, etc. rather than commercial, canned, refined white flour, sugar products and other highly processed goods in the center aisles.

Dr. Kellogg's Famous Menus:

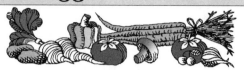

Menu #1

Breakfast

Organic Natural Sun-Dried Apricots* topped with
Raw Wheat Germ and
Sliced Banana, Pear or Orange (if desired)
(*soak in jar overnight in distilled water or
unsweetened pineapple juice)

OR

you may substitute any morning the
Bragg Healthy Energy Smoothie Drink on page 114
for a delicious energy breakfast. Remember to earn
your breakfast with doing some exercise first.

Lunch

Organic Raw Vegetable Combination Salad
Grated Raw Beet, Carrot, Turnip, Zucchini,
Chopped Tomato, Cabbage, Green Onions and
Sprouts: Alfalfa, Mung or Sunflower

Healthy Salad Dressing
Fresh Lemon or Orange, Bragg Olive Oil, dab of honey
or try Bragg's delicious Salad Dressings & Marinades
(see pages 216-217)

$^1/4$ Cup of Raw Sunflower or Pumpkin Seeds
(rich in Protein and Natural Oil)

Raw Apple

Dinner

Organic Green-Leaf Variety Salad
with Raw Mixed Lettuces and Spinach, Kale, Cucumber,
Carrot, Celery, Tomato, Parsley or Watercress

Protein – Tofu or Cooked Brown Rice
with Beans or Lentils *(Recipe on page 115)*

Fresh Fruit

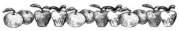

Organic apples daily helps keep the doctor away!
Apples give you Vitamin C – a powerful antioxidant and pectin, a
soluble fiber that can help lower cholesterol and glucose (sugar) levels!

Dr. Kellogg's Famous Menus:

Menu #2

Breakfast

Apple Sauce*
Steel Cut Oats – hot cereal**
served with Honey, Blackstrap Molasses,
Pure Maple Syrup or Stevia (page 177)
100% Whole Wheat or Rye Toast
(*Make your own Apple Sauce, if desired add Honey)
(**Top and serve with Sliced Ripe Banana or other Fruit)

Lunch

Organic Raw Vegetable Combination Salad
(Same as Menu #1)
Vegetable Soup with Natural Barley and Lentils
Whole Rye Toast or Oat Bran-Raisin Muffin

113

Dinner

Cabbage, Apple & Carrot Coleslaw with Spring Onions
Brown Rice or Baked Potato with Skin
Baked or Steamed Carrots and Peas
Fresh Fruit OR
Avocado, Red Onion and Tomato Salad
Steamed Asparagus or Broccoli
Raw Nuts and Seeds of any kind
Fresh Fruit

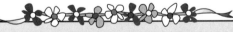

Eat Plenty of Cabbage: Miracle Cleanser & Healer

Cabbage (raw) has amazing properties. It stimulates immune system, kills bacteria and viruses, and helps heal ulcers. According to Dr. James Balch in "Prescription for Cooking and Dietary Wellness", your chances of contracting colon cancer can be reduced by up to 60% by eating cabbage weekly. Dr. Saxon-Graham states, those who never consumed cabbage were 3 times more likely to develop colon cancer. A Japanese study shows that people who ate cabbage had the lowest fatality rate from any cancer. Therapeutic benefits have also been attributed to cabbage in relation to scurvy, gout, rheumatism (arthritis), eye diseases, asthma, pyorrhea and gangrene. See our Bragg Salad Recipe (page 115). We love raw cabbage and also make a variety of sandwiches wrapped in cabbage leaves instead of bread. Try doing this – so delicious!

These freshly squeezed organic vegetable and fruit juices are important to The Bragg Healthy Lifestyle. It's not wise to drink beverages with your main meals, as it dilutes the digestive juices. But it's great during the day to have a glass of freshly squeezed orange, grapefruit, vegetable juice, Bragg Vinegar ACV Drink, herb tea or try hot cup Bragg Liquid Aminos Broth ($^{1}/_{2}$ to 1 tsp. Bragg Liquid Aminos in cup of hot distilled water) – these are all ideal pick-me-up beverages.

Bragg Apple Cider Vinegar Cocktail – Mix 1 to 2 tsps. Bragg Organic ACV and (*optional*) to taste raw honey, agave nectar or pure maple syrup in 8 oz. of distilled or purified water. Take glass upon arising, hour before lunch and dinner (*if diabetic, to sweeten use 2 stevia drops*). Bragg Organic ACV drinks now available in 6 fruit flavors, see page 218.

Delicious Hot or Cold Cider Drink – Add 2 to 3 cinnamon sticks and 4 cloves to water and boil. Steep 20 minutes or more. Before serving add Bragg Vinegar and sweetener to taste (*Re-use cinnamon sticks & cloves*).

Bragg Favorite Juice Cocktail – This drink consists of all raw vegetables (please remember organic is best) which we prepare in our vegetable juicer: carrots, celery, beets, cabbage, tomatoes, watercress and parsley, etc. The great purifier, garlic we enjoy, but it's optional.

114

Bragg Favorite Healthy Energy Smoothie – After morning stretch and exercises we often enjoy this drink instead of fruit. It's delicious and powerfully nutritious as a meal anytime: lunch, dinner or take in thermos to work, school, sports, gym, hiking, and to park or freeze for popsicles.

Bragg Healthy Energy Smoothie

Prepare following in blender, add frozen juice cube if desired colder; Choice of: freshly squeezed orange or grapefruit juice; carrot and greens juice; unsweetened pineapple juice; or $1^{1}/_{2}$ - 2 cups purified or distilled water with:

2 tsps spirulina or green powder	*1 to 2 bananas, ripe*
$^{1}/_{3}$ tsp Bragg Nutritional Yeast	*or fresh fruit in season*
2 dates or prunes, pitted (optional)	*$^{1}/_{2}$ tsp lecithin granules*
1 "Emergen-C" Vitamin C packet	*1 tsp soy protein powder*
1-2 tsps organic almond or nut butter	*1 tsp raw honey (optional)*
$^{1}/_{2}$ tsp flax seed oil or grind seeds	*$^{1}/_{2}$ tsp rice or oat bran*

Optional: 4 apricots (sundried, unsulphured) soak in jar overnight in purified/distilled water or unsweetened pineapple juice. We soak enough to last for several days. Keep refrigerated. In summer you can add organic fresh fruit: peaches, papaya, blueberries, strawberries, all berries, apricots, etc. instead of banana. In winter, add apples, kiwi, oranges, tangelos, persimmons or pears, and if fresh is unavailable, try sugar-free, frozen organic fruits. Serves 1 to 2.

Patricia's Delicious Health Popcorn

Use freshly popped organic popcorn (use air popper). Try Bragg Organic Olive Oil or flax seed oil or melted salt-free butter over popcorn and add several sprays of Bragg Liquid Aminos and Bragg Apple Cider Vinegar – Yes, it's delicious! Now sprinkle with Bragg Nutritional Yeast Seasoning and Bragg Sprinkle (24 herbs & spices). For a variety try a pinch of cayenne pepper, mustard powder or fresh crushed garlic to oil mixture. Serve instead of breads!

Bragg Lentil & Brown Rice Casserole, Burgers or Soup
Jack LaLanne's Favorite Recipe

14 oz pkg lentils, uncooked
3 carrots, chop 1" rounds
2 celery stalks, chop, (optional)
1 onion, chop, (optional)
5-6 cups, distilled /purified water

$1^1/_2$ cups brown organic rice, uncooked
4 garlic cloves, chop, (optional)
1 tsp Bragg Liquid Aminos
$^1/_4$ tsp Bragg Sprinkle (24 Herbs & Spices)
2 tsps Bragg Organic Virgin Olive Oil

Wash & drain lentils & rice. Place grains in large stainless steel pot. Add water, bring to boil, reduce to medium heat. Last 20 minutes add veggies & seasonings to grains. If desired, last 5 minutes add fresh or can (salt-free) tomatoes. For delicious garnish add spray of Bragg Aminos, minced parsley & Bragg Nutritional Yeast Seasoning. Mash or blend for burgers. For soup, add more water. Serves 4 to 6.

Bragg Raw Organic Vegetable Health Salad

2 stalks celery, chop
1 bell pepper & seeds, dice
$^1/_2$ cucumber, slice
2 carrots, grate
1 raw beet, grate
1 cup green cabbage, chop

$^1/_2$ cup red cabbage, chop
$^1/_2$ cup alfalfa or sunflower sprouts
2 spring onions & green tops, chop
1 turnip, grate
1 avocado (ripe)
3 tomatoes, medium size

For variety add organic raw zucchini, sugar peas, mushrooms, broccoli, cauliflower, (try black olives & pasta). Chop, slice or grate vegetables **115** fine to medium for variety in size. Mix vegetables & serve on bed of lettuce, spinach, watercress or chopped cabbage. Dice avocado & tomato, serve in bowl as side dressing. Serve choice of fresh squeezed lemon, orange or dressing separately. Chill salad plates before serving. **It's best to always eat salad first before serving hot dishes.** Serves 3-5.

Bragg Health Salad Dressing

$^1/_2$ cup Bragg Organic Apple Cider Vinegar
1-2 tsps organic raw honey

$^1/_2$ tsp Bragg Liquid Aminos
1-2 cloves garlic, minced

$^1/_3$ cup Bragg Organic Olive Oil, or blend with safflower, soy, sesame or flax oil
1 Tbsp fresh herbs, minced or pinch of Bragg Sprinkle (24 herbs & spices)

Blend ingredients in blender or jar. Refrigerate in covered jar.

FOR DELICIOUS HERBAL VINEGAR: In quart jar add $^1/_3$ cup tightly packed, crushed fresh sweet basil, tarragon, dill, oregano, or any fresh herbs desired, combined or singly. (If dried herbs, use 1-2 tsps herbs.) Now cover to top with Bragg Organic Apple Cider Vinegar and store two weeks in warm place, and then strain and refrigerate vinegar.

Honey – Celery Seed Vinaigrette

$^1/_4$ tsp dry mustard
$^1/_4$ tsp Bragg Liquid Aminos
$^1/_4$ tsp paprika or to taste
1-2 Tbsps raw honey or to taste

1 cup Bragg Organic Apple Cider Vinegar
$^1/_2$ cup Bragg Organic Extra Virgin Olive Oil
$^1/_2$ small onion, minced
$^1/_3$ tsp celery seed (or vary amount to taste)

Blend ingredients in blender or jar. Refrigerate in covered jar.

BENEFITS FROM THE JOYS OF FASTING

Fasting renews your faith in yourself, your strength and God's strength.
Fasting is easier than any diet. • Fasting is the quickest way to lose weight.
Fasting is adaptable to a busy life. • Fasting gives the body a physiological rest.
Fasting is used successfully in the treatment of many physical illnesses.
Fasting can yield weight losses of up to 10 pounds or more in the first week.
Fasting lowers & normalizes cholesterol, homocysteine & blood pressure levels.
Fasting improves dietary habits. • Fasting increases pleasure eating healthy foods.
Fasting is a calming experience, often relieving tension and insomnia.
Fasting frequently induces feelings of euphoria, a natural high.
Fasting is a miracle rejuvenator, slowing the ageing process.
Fasting is a natural stimulant to rejuvenate the growth hormone levels.
Fasting is an energizer, not a debilitator. • Fasting aids the elimination process.
Fasting often results in a more vigorous marital relationship.
Fasting can eliminate smoking, drug and drinking addictions.
Fasting is a regulator, educating the body to consume food only as needed.
Fasting saves time spent marketing, preparing and eating.
Fasting rids the body of toxins, giving it an internal shower & cleansing.
Fasting does not deprive the body of essential nutrients.
Fasting can be used to uncover the sources of food allergies.
Fasting is used effectively in schizophrenia treatment & other mental illnesses.
Fasting under proper supervision can be tolerated easily up to four weeks.
Fasting does not accumulate appetite; hunger pangs disappear in 1-2 days.
Fasting is routine for most of the animal kingdom.
Fasting has been a common practice since the beginning of man's existence.
116 Fasting is a rite in all religions; the Bible alone has 74 references to fasting.
Fasting under proper conditions is absolutely safe. • Fasting is a blessing.
Fasting As A Way Of Life – Allan Cott, M.D.
Fasting is not starving, it's nature's cure that God has given us. – Patricia Bragg

Spiritual Bible Reasons Why We Should Fast

Acts 13:2-3	Neh. 1:4	Luke 4:2-5, 14	Deut. 8:3-8	Matthew 9:9-15
Acts 14:23-25	Ezra 8:21	Luke 9:1-6, 11	Joel 2:12	Matthew 17:18-21
3 John 2	Gal. 5:16-26	Mark 2:16-20	Matthew 7:7-8	Deut. 11:7-14, 21
1 Cor. 10:31	Gen. 6:3	Matthew 4:1-4	Psalms 119:18	Neh. 9:1, 20-21
1 Cor. 13:4-7	Isaiah 58:6, 8	Psalms 69:10	Psalms 35:13	Matthew 6:16-18

Dear Health Friend,

This gentle reminder explains the great benefits from *The Miracle of Fasting* that you will enjoy when starting on your weekly 24 hour Bragg Fasting Program for Super Health! It's a precious time of body-mind-soul cleansing and renewal.

On fast days I drink 8-10 glasses of distilled (our favorite) or purified water, (I add 1-2 tsps Bragg Organic Vinegar to 3 of them). If just starting, you may also try herbal teas or try diluted fresh juices with $^1/_3$ distilled water. Every day, even some fast days, add 1 Tbsp of psyllium husk powder to liquids once daily. It's an extra cleanser and helps normalize weight, cholesterol and blood pressure and helps promote healthy elimination. Fasting is the oldest, most effective healing method known to man. Fasting offers great, miraculous blessings from Mother Nature and our Creator. It begins the self-cleansing of the inner-body workings so we can promote our own self-healing.

My father and I wrote the book *The Miracle of Fasting* to share with you the health miracles it can perform in your life. It's all so worthwhile to do and it's an important part of The Bragg Healthy Lifestyle.

With Love, *Patricia*

Paul Bragg's work on fasting and water is one of the great contributions to The Healing Wisdom and The Natural Health Movement in the world today.

– Gabriel Cousens, M.D., Author of *Conscious Eating & Spiritual Nutrition*

Chapter 7

Exercise

Fourth Step Towards Building Nerve Force

There is nothing better to build powerful Nerve Force than a brisk two to five mile hike everyday. You're too old and flabby? Nonsense! Dad's a great, great grandfather and he loves to hike, jog, run, swim, ride his bicycle, climb mountains, play tennis and enjoys playing many other athletic sports. You're never too old to start! Of course, we don't expect you to plunge right in and become an athlete overnight! Do it gradually. Start out with a one mile hike every day for a week. Then increase it to two miles. As you exercise your muscles, your blood starts circulating briskly through your body. Breathe deeply and fill your lungs with oxygen. You will feel new vigor and vitality surging through you! You will eat with a good appetite and you will sleep like a baby. Your Nerve Force reservoirs will soon be filled with energy, go-power and you will have a new zest for living! **117**

The more time you spend in the fresh air and gentle sunshine doing physical activity, the greater your reserves of Nerve Force will be! In our long experience as teachers of health, fitness and longevity, we found those who exercise regularly have greater poise and a more balanced personality. They are also generally free from nervous and emotional stress that plague the typically inactive person. This is apparent among children. The inactive child who refuses to join his playmates in play, games and sports is generally the "odd" child, nervous and emotionally unstable. The active child who loves playing games and sports is almost always better balanced emotionally because their energies are directed along constructive lines of action. The same holds true with teenagers. When their energies are channeled into games, sports and outdoor activities, children don't have idle time or energy to get in trouble. They enjoy better grades, health and family togetherness.

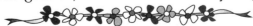

Exercise, aerobics, walking, biking, rollerblading, swimming, jogging, tennis and most all sports benefit your body and brain power and helps you think faster. Studies show exercise keeps the brain younger and helps retain the quick response of youth.

In the Hawaiian Islands, the swimming is so ideal that Hawaii has great fun hosting swimming contests with youngsters of all ages. They splash and dive in the water, and their merry laughter rings in the clear, tropical air! When we talk to the parents of these active children, we find they have absolutely no emotional or social problems with them. No matter what your age, exercise can do wonders for you! It is never too late to start tapping the rich veins of vitality lying dormant within every person! If you want to be well-balanced emotionally and free of stresses, strains and tensions – make it a habit to get outdoors for physical activity at least once every day.

Walk Off Your Emotional Tensions

We learned many years ago that we could actually walk off our emotional strains. No matter how serious the problems we faced, we could find the answer to our dilemma in a brisk two mile walk. Some of the greatest decisions we have had to make in our lives were made during one of our hikes. As the oxygen floods into the body from vigorous walking, one can think more clearly.

A wealthy friend telephoned Dad during the great financial depression of the 1930s and said, "Paul, I am completely ruined financially. I am going to kill myself, and I called up to say good-bye." My father asked this tormented man to grant him just one favor. When he agreed, Dad said, "All right, we will have a walk and a farewell talk before you end your life."

Dad got in his car, dashed to his friend's home and off they went, hiking for a full five hours. During that time father told him that money was not the only thing in life and that he had to get some perspective and straighten out his values. Dad literally walked some sense into him! Had that man stayed at home and brooded over his loses, he would have destroyed himself, but that long nature walk in fresh air changed his whole life! Dad's friend was not rich materially, but rich in inner wealth.

Our friend, engineer Jim Cotton, back in 1969 started the "Waikiki Rough Water Swim Series" and dad enjoyed being in this event. Now there's over 3,000 yearly in this popular 2 mile rough water swim. Dr. John Westerdahl, Bragg's Health Institute Director has participated in this swim yearly.

Expert Advice on How to Exercise

Often you may ask yourself, "why aren't you closing in on your ideal weight?" You're trying to workout and exercise, but your bathroom scale is not showing you any results – your weight appears the same as when you started out. Here are some tips from the experts:

(1) An effective weekly exercise program should get your heart pumping. Include one rigorous program that makes you sweat; two moderate exercise programs, and one easy session. For example: take an aerobics or Zumba workout class and then a more relaxing yoga class.

(2) Drink at least 64 ounces (2 quarts) of purified water daily. Drinking water has a huge effect on exercise. Dehydrated exercisers worked out 25% less effectively than those who drank water before and during workouts.

(3) In the initial phases of the exercise training, you may get post-workout dips in blood sugar that cause cravings for simple carbohydrates like sweets, etc. these cravings should disappear a few weeks into your exercise training. It's wise to have the Bragg Vinegar Drink, fresh fruits (apple, banana, orange, etc.), or some trail mix available to prevent reaching for a candy bar.

119

What Miracles Exercise Can Do for You

Get outdoors fast and get physically active when you feel dark moods, anxieties, worries, blues, depression and tensions overtaking you – otherwise these negative moods can damage you! Walking or any other outdoor exercise will help clear up your thinking and put your problems in perspective. Any form of outdoor recreation recreates the human personality. The ancient men of India who desired to become one with God believed the body and bloodstream had to be pure and strong before this could become a reality. Thus, they developed a physical fitness system called Yoga. They daily practice their belief that the body is meant to be stretched, strengthened and exercised correctly in order to remain healthy. No matter what your calendar years, start turning back your biological clock now faithfully with exercise.

If I had to pick one thing . . . that comes closest to
the Fountain of Youth, it would be exercise!
– Dr. James Fries, M.D., expert on ageing at Stanford University

Benefits that Moderate Daily Exercise Brings You:

1 Exercise increases circulation, and brings more oxygen into your body. You will feel more energetic.

2 Exercise relieves stress, strain and tension. Tension gets locked in the tight, stiffened areas of your body, especially the neck, back and spine. Exercise will stretch and loosen these areas as it restores youthful limberness. You will feel more relaxed and at ease.

3 Overcoming chronic tiredness is a major benefit of exercise. That chronic tired feeling to a great extent is due to a lack of sufficient circulation to your brain. Exercise brings the oxygen-laden blood into this vital area with an energizing and revitalizing effect.

4 Exercise helps calm the nerves. Nothing can calm the nerves better than 30 minutes of brisk walking and exercise. It also helps to promote a good night's sleep, which is absolutely essential to maintaining calmness, repose, serenity and health.

5 Exercise increases emotional control. Exercise helps to strengthen the nerves of the body and helps create the healthy composure that comes from a healthy nervous system and a balanced, happy state of mind.

Exercise Promotes Health & Youthfulness

We know that healthy living with proper exercise can produce a new breed of men and women who will enjoy more strength to carry out their daily work and have sufficient energy left for after-work interests, family and hobbies. They can retain the prime of life for 20 to 40 years longer than the person who is lazy and will not exercise! Examples: both Tom Selleck and Clint Eastwood exercise, lift weights and eat healthy.

All external characteristics of health (such as powerful Nerve Force) are but the result of the healthy functioning of your vital internal organs and glands. These are what keep you going. Exercise actually reaches into your body bringing about miracle improvements in certain internal parts such as your nervous system, your heart, liver, lungs, kidneys, entire digestive tract, colon and thyroid gland among others. To attain these benefits you should faithfully follow a regular program of exercise.

Is age a hindrance to daily exercise? The answer is unequivocally, "No"! In fact, age is no excuse for not exercising! Our friend Roy White, 106 years young, walked 3 to 8 miles daily! (page 60). No one is too old to continue safe exercise! Conrad Hilton jogged daily to almost 100.

To rest is to rust! It is far better to wear out than to rust out. The saying, *If you don't use it, you lose it,* certainly applies to the 640 muscles of the body. When you don't exercise regularly, your muscles lose their supple tone. As soon as you put down this book go outdoors and take a brisk, invigorating walk. Say out loud while walking: *Health! Peace! Joy! Love for Eternity!* You will feel great and your trillions of cells will rejoice with circulation!

Enjoy Exercising – It's Healthy and Fun!

There is great hiking near where we had a home in Hollywood, California, where Mt. Hollywood rises some 2,000 feet in famous Griffith Park. We enjoyed early morning hikes up the mountain to greet the sun rising and then run down. Also, in Santa Barbara, CA, we always enjoy an ocean swim and hiking in the surrounding foothills.

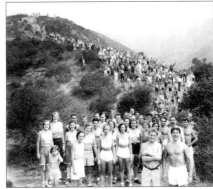

A thousand Happy Bragg Health Students enjoy hiking, exercise and fresh air on the trail to Mt. Hollywood, CA, summer, 1932.

121

We love to walk, jog and climb mountains. We make time to walk or jog daily, or we swim, play tennis or ride our bikes. We work out 3 times a week with a progressive weight training program, which helps keep our bones and muscles healthier and stronger. See pages 123 to 124.

Exercise is the greatest single health factor available to us that helps us remove any blockages and unclog the arteries and blood vessels, and for increasing the vital flow of oxygen-enriched blood throughout the heart and body! Recent studies show that exercise improves health and also reduces the risk of developing adult-onset diabetes as well as breast cancer. The Harvard School of Public Health Researchers (*www.health.harvard.edu*) studied 70,000 women. Results: 46% lowered their risk of diabetes with daily vigorous exercising and brisk walking.

Enjoy Exercise & Jogs for Longer Life

On our world Bragg Health Crusades the first question we ask the hotel manager is, where is the nearest park where we can take our daily exercise? And off we go sometime during the day. We prefer to go early in the morning or late in the afternoon. Each person, however, should choose the time best suited and available to them.

We are so pleased to find that all over the world today walking, hiking, running and jogging have become an accepted method in the pursuit of Heart Fitness by people of all age groups. Many cities have walking, hiking and jogging clubs (*www.joggers.co.nz, TheWalkingSite.com* and *SierraClub.com*). We have enjoyed running with folks world-wide; including Europe, England, Australia, New Zealand and throughout the USA.

It's universally accepted exercise is important for physical, mental and emotional health. A daily run or jog when adapted to individual's physical condition and age will improve endurance, produce sense of well-being and help to maintain total body fitness (each step gives your trillions of cells a massage, also try trampolining and stationary jogging while watching TV). Exercise helps increase resistance to sickness and disease, and helps make the heart stronger and life longer!

122

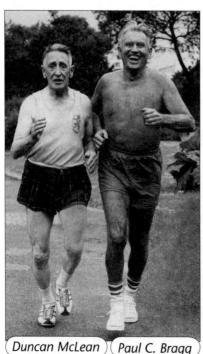

Duncan McLean   Paul C. Bragg

Before starting on your exercise program, it's wise to seek advice from your health practitioner. Also, be sure that you choose a soft surface to run or jog on, such as grass or sand. Jogging on hard surfaces, such as concrete and asphalt, could accumulate damage to your knees, hips, ankles and other organs.

Bragg with friend Duncan McLean, England's oldest Champion Sprinter, (83 years young) on a training run in London's beautiful Regent's Park.

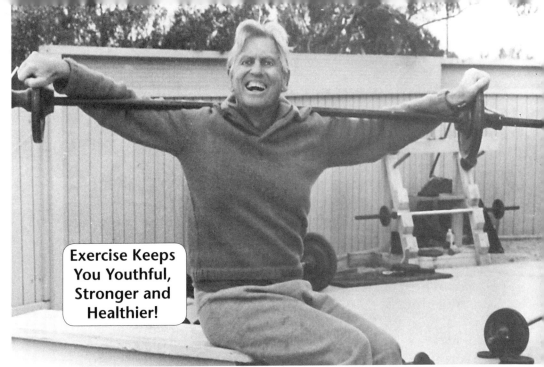

Paul C. Bragg and Patricia lift weights 3 times weekly.

Iron-Pumping Oldsters (ages 86 to 96) Triple Their Muscle Strength In Landmark U.S. Government Study

WASHINGTON NEWS — Ageing nursing home residents in Boston *pumping iron?* Elderly weightlifters tripling and quadrupling their muscle strength? Is it possible? Most people would doubt and wonder at this amazing revelation! (Website study listed on page 124.)

Yet the government experts on ageing answered those questions with resounding *"yes"* according to results of this study. They turned a group of frail Boston nursing home residents, aged 86 to 96, into weightlifters to demonstrate that it's never too late to reverse age-related declines in muscle strength. The study group participated in a regime of high-intensity weight-training research conducted by the Agriculture Departments Human Research Center of Ageing at Tufts University in Boston. *A high-intensity weight training program is capable of inducing dramatic increases in the muscle strength in frail men and women up to 96 years of age.* This was reported by Dr. Maria A. Fiatarone, who was the Study Director.

The favorable response to strength training in these subjects was remarkable in light of their very advanced age, extremely sedentary habits, many chronic diseases, functional disabilities and nutritional inadequacies.

Despite their many handicaps, the elderly weight lifters increased their muscle strength by 3 to 4 times in as little as 8 weeks. Dr. Fiatarone said they were stronger at the program's end than they had been in years!

See web: *antiagingresearch.com/behavioral_factors.shtml*

Fiatarone and her associates emphasized the safety of such a closely supervised weight lifting program, even among people in frail health. The average age of the 10 participants was 90. Six had coronary heart disease, 7 had arthritis, 6 had bone fractures resulting from osteoporosis, 4 had high blood pressure, and all had been physically inactive for years. Yet no serious medical problems resulted from this program. A few of the participants did report minor muscle and joint aches, but 9 of the 10 still completed the program.

The study participants, drawn from a 712 bed long-term care facility in Boston, worked out 3 times a week during the study. They performed 3 sets of 8 repetitions with each leg on a weight lifting machine. The weights were gradually increased from 10 pounds to about 40 pounds at the end of the 8 week program.

Fiatarone said the study carries potentially important implications for older people, who represent a growing proportion of the population. A decline in muscle strength and size is one of the more predictable features of ageing! Muscle strength in the average adult decreases by 30% to 50% during the course of a lifetime. Experts on ageing do not know whether the decrease is an unavoidable consequence of ageing, or results mainly from sedentary lifestyle and other controllable factors.

Exercise, along with healthy foods and some fasting helps maintain or restore a healthy physical balance and normal weight for a long, happy life.

Exercise is the Best Fitness Conditioner

A daily program of walking, running or jogging is a quick, sure and inexpensive fitness conditioner. Be faithful to your exercise routine for true heart fitness. Women will be especially pleased when they see fat change to lean, as the inches fly off their waistlines and hiplines – all the while improving their health! Men and women, both please remember your waistline is your lifeline and also your dateline! A person with a trim and fit figure always looks more youthful and attractive!

If you are a *softie* and feel you cannot get outside for your run or jog on cold and rainy days – stationary inside jogging to music or your favorite talk show will work too. Stay in one place and lift one foot at a time about 6-8 inches from floor – it's best to start easy and gradually build up to faster, longer periods. Remember to exercise where you get the most fresh air – on the patio, front porch, or inside or outside rest areas at work.

The Miracle Life of Ageless Jack LaLanne

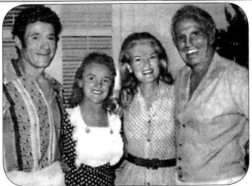

Jack LaLanne, Patricia Bragg, Elaine LaLanne & Paul C. Bragg

Jack says he would have been dead by 16 if he hadn't attended The Bragg Crusade. Jack says, *Bragg saved my life at age 15, when I attended the Bragg Health and Fitness Crusade in Oakland, California.* From that day on, Jack has continued to live The Bragg Healthy Lifestyle, inspiring millions to health, fitness and a long fulfilled, happy life! See Jack LaLanne's great web: *jacklalanne.com*

It's proven that exercise helps, but over 60% of U.S. adults do not get enough physical activity to help keep them healthy and fit.

For instant mood lifter, take a brisk walk and count your blessings. Exercise and fresh air has positive effects on the human spirit and mind.

Macfadden – Founder of Physical Culture

Macfadden was the father of Physical Culture in America and Paul C. Bragg the father of the Health Movement and the originator of Health Food Stores. Paul Bragg began his lifetime career in Natural Physical Fitness early in the last century by working with famous Physical Culture pioneer, Bernarr Macfadden. Bragg was editor of Macfadden's Physical Culture Magazine, the first publication to bring the basic principles of healthful living to popular attention in America. They were credited with "getting women out of bloomers into shorts, and men into bathing trunks." Bragg started Macfadden's "Penny Kitchen Restaurants" during the big Depression Era, when they fed millions of hungry people for a penny each. Bragg helped develop America's first Health Spa at Dansville, New York, where this photo was taken. Bragg then opened Macfadden's Deauville Hotel, which gave undeveloped Miami Beach, Florida its great beginning.

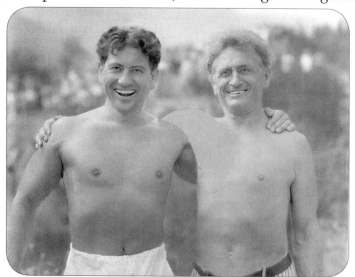

Paul C. Bragg & Mentor – Bernarr Macfadden

My dad was associated with Bernarr Macfadden, who spent thousands of dollars to find the *oldest living humans* on earth. Dad was his main researcher on this project. This took him to many interesting, remote parts of the world, interviewing men and women from *103 to 154 years of age!* Dad found this work fascinating, because he loved promoting health and longevity, that not just the life of the average person which ends at about 70-72, but an active life that would last 120 to 150 years (Genesis 6:3). The Bragg research proved it can be done! Now Scientists worldwide are agreeing.

20 Year Study Shows Being Fit Saves Money

The average American spends over $4,000 on health care yearly, and costs are rising: Private health-insurance premiums jumped 8.2% even back in 1998, more than double the previous years (3.3% in 1996, 3.5% in 1997) and way up in 2011. This revealing 20 year study done by Dr. Tedd Mitchell of Cooper Clinic in Texas monitored 6,679 men. Results showed those who exercised more, required fewer doctor visits. Being fit cuts yearly medical expenses 25 to 60%. Study also found all you need to stay fit is to exercise just 20 to 30 minutes a day, four or five days a week. Physically fit people live longer and enjoy a better quality of life! Visit website: *cooperwellness.com*

The Benefits of Being Fit & Healthy

The benefits of being fit and keeping active, is an improved quality of life – being able to do things you enjoy for longer periods of time. To be fit, one must have good habits! This includes eating healthy foods like organic fruits and vegetables, exercising regularly, getting enough sleep and being clean. Becoming fit will help you tremendously both physically and mentally. As you become more fit these benefits will happen:

Looking Better: weight loss, toned muscles, better posture

Feeling Better: more energy, better sleep, better able to cope with stress, reduced depression and anxiety, increased mental sharpness, and fewer aches and pains

Being Healthier: more efficient heart and lungs, lower cholesterol, lower blood pressure, ability to heal faster, stronger bones with less risk of osteoporosis, less stress on your joints, better balance and flexibility, strengthened immune system, and reduced risk of dying early, heart disease, obesity, diabetes, cancers, stroke, etc. (*icb2001.com*)

Exercising just 15 minutes or more a day helps maintain healthy blood vessels for good circulation in the body and brain and helps you manage your weight and stress levels. Studies have shown that brisk walking helps delay brain shrinkage that delays the onset of dementia.

Healthy Heart Habits for a Long, Vital Life

Remember, *organic live foods make live people. You are what you eat, drink, breathe, think, say and do.* So eat a low-fat, low-sugar, high-fiber diet of organic whole grains, fresh salads, sprouts, greens, vegetables, fruits, raw seeds, nuts, fresh juices and chemical-free, purified or distilled water.

Earn your food with daily exercise, for regular exercise, brisk walking, etc. improves your health, stamina, go-power, flexibility, endurance and helps open the cardiovascular system. Only 45 minutes a day truly can do miracles for your heart, arteries, mind, nerves, soul and body! You become revitalized with new zest for living to accomplish your life goals!

We are made of tubes. To help keep them open, clean and to maintain good elimination take fiber capsule or add 1 tsp psyllium husk powder or oat bran daily – hour after dinner to juices, herbal teas, even Bragg Vinegar Drink. Another way to guard against clogged tubes daily – add 1-2 tsps soy lecithin granules (*fat emulsifier-melts like butter*) over potatoes, veggies and to juices, etc. Also take one cayenne capsule (40,000 HU) daily with meal. Take 50-100 mgs regular-released niacin (B3) with one meal daily to help cleanse and open cardiovascular system, also improves memory. Skin flushing may occur, don't worry about this as it shows it's working! After cholesterol level reaches 180, then only take niacin twice weekly.

The heart needs healthy balanced nutrients, so take natural multi-vitamin-mineral food supplements, Omega-3 and extra heart helpers – vitamin E with mixed Tocotrienols, vitamin C, Ubiquinol CoQ10, D3, MSM, D-Ribose, garlic, turmeric, selenium, zinc, beta carotene and amino acids: L-Carnitine, L-Taurine, L-Lysine and Proline. Folic acid, CoQ10, B6 and B12 helps keep homocysteine level low. Magnesium Orotate, Hawthorn Berry Extract helps bring relief for palpitations, arrhythmia, senile hearts and coronary disease. Braggzyme contains systemic enzymes (nattokinase & serrapetase) to help keep blood thin, preventing dangerous blood clots. Take multi-digestive enzyme and probiotics with meals – aids digestion, assimilation and elimination.

For sleep problems try 5-HTP Tryptophan (an amino acid), melatonin, calcium, magnesium, valerian in caps, extract or tea, Bragg vinegar drink & sleepytime herb tea. For arthritis, joint pain/stiffness, try Braggzyme, aloe juice & gel, Glucosamine - Chondroitin - MSM combo caps or shots, helps heal & regenerate. Capsaicin & DMSO lotion helps relieve pain.

Use amazing antioxidants – E Tocotrienols, C, Quercetin, grapeseed extract (OPCs), CoQ10, selenium, SOD, Resveratrol, Alpha-Lipoic Acid, etc. They improve immune system and help flush out dangerous free radicals that cause havoc with cardiovascular pipes and health. Research shows antioxidants promote longevity, slows ageing, fights toxins, helps prevent disease, cancer, cataracts, jet lag and exhaustion.

128

Recommended Heart Health Tests

- **Total Cholesterol:** Adults: 180 mg/dl is optimal; **Children:** 140 mg/dl or less
- **LDL Cholesterol:** 100 mg/dl or less is optimal
- **HDL Cholesterol:** Men: 50 mg/dl or more; **Women:** 65 mg/dl or more
- **Triglycerides:** 100 mg/dl or less (optimal 70-85)
- **HDL/Cholesterol Ratio:** 3.2 or less • **Triglycerides/HDL Ratio:** below 2
- **Homocysteine:** 6-8 micromoles/L
- **CRP (C-Reactive Protein high sensitivity):**
  lower than 1 mg/L low risk, 1-3 mg/L average risk, over 3 mg/L high risk
- **Diabetic Risk Tests:** • **Glucose:** 80-100 mg/dl • **Hemoglobin A1c:** 7% or less
- **Blood Pressure:** 120/70 mmHg is considered optimal for adults

Chapter 8

Correct Breathing

Fifth Step Towards Powerful Nerve Force

Oxygen-starved people are usually nervous people with many problems. As we have discussed, the activity of the vital organs depends directly upon the nerve stimulus they receive from the nervous system. Nerve Exhaustion therefore impairs the action of the stomach, kidneys, bowels and other abdominal organs, causing digestive distress and other innumerable ailments.

The heart and lungs are especially affected by Nerve Exhaustion and nerve tension! We all have observed that the slightest excitement will speed up our heart beat and breathing. Fear and worry depress the action of the heart and lungs, an effect which can become quite serious. The heart and lungs – upon which life depends more directly than any other organs – may be considered the master organs of the body. When the heart stops beating, death will result in a few minutes, and the heart will stop beating soon after its oxygen supply is shut off.

129

The blood is your river of life and it must be kept pure! It is one of the main duties of the heart and lungs to do this important task. With each breath, life-giving oxygen is carried into the blood, while deadly poisonous carbon dioxide is transported away.

Deep Breathers Live Longer

Air is the body's most important energizer. The more deeply you breathe pure air, the better your chances are for extending your life. For over 75 years, we have done extensive research on long-lived people and we've discovered this common denominator: they are all deep breathers. We have found that the deeper, fewer breaths a person takes in one minute, the longer they live. Most rapid breathers are short-lived. It's essential and life-enhancing that we breathe deeply and correctly for super health.

Oxygen is the main nutrient of the body. When we improve our oxygen intake by exercising and deep breathing, we enhance our immune system and the body's ability to detoxify and stay healthy.
– Dr. Michael Schachter, Columbia University

The Lower Respiratory System

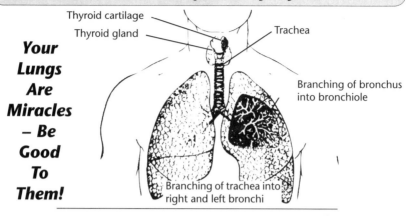

Your Lungs Are Miracles – Be Good To Them!

Thyroid cartilage

Thyroid gland

Trachea

Branching of bronchus into bronchiole

Branching of trachea into right and left bronchi

Path of Breath

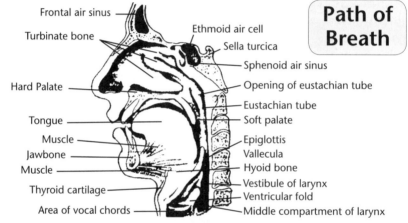

Frontal air sinus

Turbinate bone

Hard Palate

Tongue

Muscle

Jawbone

Muscle

Thyroid cartilage

Area of vocal chords

Ethmoid air cell

Sella turcica

Sphenoid air sinus

Opening of eustachian tube

Eustachian tube

Soft palate

Epiglottis

Vallecula

Hyoid bone

Vestibule of larynx

Ventricular fold

Middle compartment of larynx

130

Mechanics of Breathing

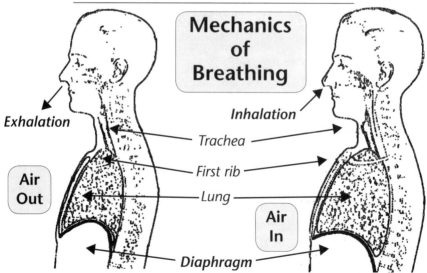

Exhalation

Air Out

Inhalation

Trachea

First rib

Lung

Air In

Diaphragm

Mechanics of Breathing, showing diaphragm position and flexible ribs at exhalation and at inhalation.

Two Methods of Breathing

There are two principal methods of breathing – Chest and Diaphragmatic Breathing. The curved line represents the diaphragm, the broad muscle which separates the heart and lungs from the abdominal organs. When this muscle contracts – moving downward – it produces suction within the chest cavity which causes an inflow of air into the lungs (inhalation). When the diaphragm rises, air is forced out of the lungs (exhalation). The alternate rise and fall of this muscle produces a corresponding movement of the abdominal organs causing the abdomen to expand and contract. This produces an alternate high and low pressure within the abdominal cavity. Diaphragmatic breathing is the proper method of tranquil breathing and may be termed *normal breathing*. This is the way babies and children naturally breathe.

Chest Breathing

It may seem strange that the breathing – which we do our whole lives – could be done incorrectly. We can observe few people breathe diaphragmatically all the time. Instead, they usually breathe by the chest method. This is because – as we become adults – the tight clothing we wear and the cramped positions we assume when sitting restrict the action of the diaphragm and compel the more powerful chest muscles to come to the rescue. This gradually instills the habit of chest breathing. Years of this practice creates a habit so deep-seated that daily faithful effort is required to correct it.

Chest breathing results from the movement of the rib section of the trunk and especially the upper section of the chest. During inhalation the chest expands and during exhalation it contracts. This form of breathing – especially when performed to the limit of inhalation and exhalation – is an excellent form of internal exercise that develops the size of the chest and is beneficial in many ways. Chest breathing is naturally employed by the body only during strenuous exertion. It might be termed a form of "forced breathing," just as a forced drought may be applied to a boiler when great steam pressure is needed.

Diaphragmatic Breathing

Diaphragmatic breathing – sometimes called "abdominal breathing" is entirely different in action from chest breathing. During inhalation the abdomen expands (becomes larger) and during exhalation the abdomen contracts (becomes smaller). It must be understood that air does not enter the abdominal region with this form of breathing. This is impossible.

How to Practice Diaphragmatic Breathing

It's best to begin practicing diaphragmatic breathing while lying down since it's more easily performed in this position. After faithfully practicing for a few weeks lying down, then do your regular practice while you are sitting or standing. Continue your conscious diaphragmatic breathing until full control is attained naturally over the diaphragm and it becomes an unconscious habit.

Conscious diaphragmatic breathing is of great help in restoring the heart action to normal. Heart fluttering, skipping of beats and other abnormal manifestations in heart action are very common in people with damaged nerves. We know of many cases in which diaphragmatic breathing helped correct the most serious forms of so-called "heart trouble". The habit of diaphragmatic breathing should be acquired as quickly as possible . . . because it is a primary requisite for Supreme Health, whether or not one is the victim of "nerves".

Advantages of Diaphragmatic Breathing

1. It promotes greater oxygenation of the blood because the air is compelled to enter mainly into the lower and larger sections of the lungs.
2. Stimulation of blood circulation in the abdominal cavity due to the breaths alternating high and low pressure in that region is essential to promote the healthy proper action of all the vital body organs.

Quick Tip: *To avoid environmental toxins that overload your immune system – eat only organic foods, stop smoking and don't hang out with anyone who does and get safe sun exposure to boost Vitamin D3 levels.*

To relax quickly, take some good deep breaths and then slowly exhale.

③ Stimulation of peristalsis – the worm-like motion of the intestines – which promotes digestion and then the elimination of toxic fecal wastes. We know of hundreds of cases in which a change from chest to diaphragmatic breathing helped to correct long standing conditions including chronic constipation, gas, heartburn, indigestion and liver troubles, etc.

④ A remarkably healthy calming effect upon the nerves – especially the pneumogastric nerve and the solar plexus. Diaphragmatic breathing breaks up the paralyzing nerve tension so often observed in people with super-sensitive or damaged nerves. The close relation between the pneumogastric nerve, breathing and the vital organs is demonstrated when a baby is born. In an unborn child in the womb, the vital organs are practically at a standstill. If food were in the stomach, it would not be digested, but with the first breath – the "breath of life" or the "breath of God" – the baby's entire vital machinery is set in motion! This breath means the awakening of the pneumogastric nerve and especially the solar plexus.

Control Jagged, Jumpy Nerves With Long, Slow Diaphragmatic Breathing

Many things can trigger the nerves into a heightened emotional state – worries and cares of all kinds, grief, emotional shock, stress, strain and tension. Family relationships can bring on nervous upsets. Husbands and wives who can't communicate have great emotional battles. Parents and children often find the generation gap so wide they can't bridge it and this produces frustrations. Marital or in-law problems, financial worries and sickness can all trigger an emotional upset and stress.

Here's how to restore balance to the nervous system when an emotional upset strikes you. Go to a quiet place, even if you have to go into a closet. First just sit still. Take your pulse rate. You will find it's racing. You will also find during emotional excitement you will take rapid chest breaths. (More helpful solutions next page.)

During stress or anger, we tend to inhale and hold our breath. The significant, therapeutic aspect of this breathing is the exhalation – which is at least twice the length of the inhalation. The exhalation alerts the body it can relax and resume essential peaceful body functions.

Long, Slow Diaphragmatic Breathing Leads to a Long, Peaceful, Healthy Life!

Miracles happen when you slow down your breathing. Take full diaphragmatic breaths. See how few long, slow deep breaths you can take in a minute. After a few minutes you will find your pulse rate is slower. Your nerves begin to quiet down. Instead of trying to solve your emotional problems in a state of excitement, you are now calm. This long, slow diaphragmatic breathing allows you to shift from emotionalism to logical thinking. You become master of the situation. You no longer look at your problems subjectively, but begin to take the broad, objective view. With logical and positive thinking you can find the answers to emotional problems. If you use this technique when emotional shocks hit, you'll save yourself a lot of lost Nerve Force. This slow, deep diaphragmatic breathing is a wonderful method to calm yourself and weather life's emotional upsets.

134

The shortest lived animals are those who breathe rapidly. The longest lived animals are those who take slower breaths. Many years ago we learned this secret from a Breatharian – as he was known – who lived in India. It was claimed by many that he was over 130 years of age! He looked like a well preserved man in his early 70s. He had sharp eyes and a wrinkle-free face with a happy disposition and a keen mind. He could tell you what had happened in his life 125 years ago!

He practiced long, slow diaphragmatic breathing and did it so well that he took only one full breath per minute. He was an Indian Guru, a teacher and had attained perfect bliss consciousness. He finally went to a retreat in the Himalayan Mountains. We've been told by a man who recently returned from India that this Guru was still alive and in perfect health! Dad and I are students of deep breathing and we practice it daily. We are aware of how important oxygen (the invisible staff of life) is to our well-being and to the building of our bodies' powerful Nerve Force and super health.

ATP – adenosine triphosphate – is the basic currency of life. A dip in ATP levels results in fatigue, aches and pains. One-Breath Meditation reverses falling ATP levels, injecting you with enough vigor to see you through your current project. Sit down, straighten back, inhale deeply, clearing your mind. Relax shoulders, hold breath a moment, then exhale, releasing all tension from your muscles.

Deadly Smoking – Health Hazard to Avoid – What it Does to You & Those Around You!

When people inhale deadly tobacco smoke into their miracle lungs, the protective cilia hairs filter out much of the smoke's harmful substances before it is exhaled. This means that while harmful toxins are trapped in the delicate linings of the smokers' lungs, fewer of these toxins are re-released into the air for others to breathe in. However, between a smoker's deadly puffs, the cigarette burns directly into the air. This smoke is known as "secondhand, side-stream" smoke, but it should be called "direct" smoke. Smoke that burns directly into the air is completely unfiltered and more deadly than the smokers' smoke! Stay away from all deadly smoke!

Recent studies establish that people who live or work around smokers are more likely to develop lung and sinus damage than smokers. For asthma or bronchitis sufferers, this exposure is very damaging! In addition to these dangers, "direct" smoke irritates the eyes, nose and throat and smells up everything it touches (rooms, hotels, offices, carpets, drapes, cars and everything around smoking).

For the cigarette smoker, whose miracle lungs have unfortunately become the filters protecting the body from the deadly smoke, the effects are equally – if not more – damaging. Tar begins to collect in the lungs once there is too much to be removed through the lungs' normal cleaning processes. This means the over-burdened lungs can no longer clean normal contaminants they have to deal with. Dirt inhaled into the alveoli – which is normally trapped in a layer of sticky mucus and carried out of the lungs by the wavelike motions of the tiny cilia hairs – becomes trapped and stuck in the lungs. The cilia hairs become paralyzed by tar, so the normal cleansing (drain) procedures break down and the airways become clogged. This makes the lungs resort to coughing, spitting and respiratory-breathing attacks, flu, etc. in an effort to expel the contaminated, clogging toxins, tar and mucus.

There is good news. When a person stops smoking the cilia hairs begin to heal and move again. Smokers – stop now, you begin cleansing and healing immediately!

Neurotoxins are chemicals that injure cells in the nervous system.
Some neurotoxins are mercury, alcohol, tobacco smoke and pesticides.
– Bragg Friend, Dr. Bob Martin, author Secret Nerve Cures, doctorbob.com

DEADLY SMOKING FACTS!

✝ Tobacco use and second-hand smoke will eventually kill 1/5 of developed world population: about 250 million people.

✝ Of the 50 million Americans who smoke, one third to one half will die from a smoke-related disease. All will reduce their life expectancy by an average of nine years.

✝ Smoking acts as either a stimulant or a depressant, depending upon the smoker's emotional state.

✝ The average pack-a-day smoker takes about 70,000 *hits* of nicotine each year and with 2 packs it's 140,000 *hits*.

✝ "Second hand smoke" hurts non-smokers: it speeds up the heart rate, raises blood pressure and doubles the amount of deadly carbon monoxide in their blood.

✝ Secondary smoke contains more nicotine, tar and cadmium (leading to hypertension, bronchitis and emphysema) than mainstream smoke.

 ✝ Babies born to mothers who smoke have lower body weight, smaller lungs and more health problems.

136

✝ Lung illnesses are twice as common in smokers' children.

✝ Children and teenagers make up 90% of the new smokers in the United States – and teenage smoking is on the rise!

✝ The death rate from breast cancer ranges from 25% to 75% higher among women who smoke.

✝ Female smokers may face a higher risk of lung cancer – as much as twice the risk of male smokers, according to Dr. Harvey Risch's famous study at Yale University. *www.info.med.yale.edu/eph/faculty/risch*

✝ Your body contains over 60,000 miles of blood vessels. Smoking constricts those vessels, depriving your body of the important fresh, rich oxygen it needs.

✝ Tobacco is the main introduction to more deadly drugs.

✝ Teens who smoke are far more likely to engage in other risky and life-threatening behaviors than non-smoking teens (including using other dangerous drugs, violence, gang involvement, carrying weapons, and engaging in premarital sex, which often results in pregnancy or disease).

✝ Cataracts, cancer, angina, arteriosclerosis, osteoporosis, chronic bronchitis, high blood pressure, impotence, diabetes and respiratory ailments are linked to smoking.

Heimlich Maneuver Jumpstarts the Lungs

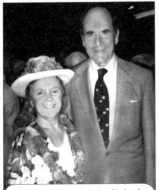

Dr. Henry J. Heimlich & Patricia Bragg in Honolulu

My father and I want to do all we can to ensure that all people are able to get the oxygen they need. We have even included how to get **asthma**, **choking** and **drowning** accident victims breathing again, page 138.

Many of you are familiar with the famous Heimlich Maneuver as a technique for saving choking victims. Since 1974, this procedure has saved over 100,000 lives just in the United States. This maneuver, developed by Dr. Henry J. Heimlich, is performed by pressing upward on the diaphragm. This compresses the lungs, causing a flow of air that helps push the choking object out that is blocking the airway. Recent evidence and research has suggested the Heimlich Maneuver is effective in restoring breathing in more emergency situations than just choking. Our friends Dr. Heimlich along with his wife Jane Murray Heimlich is, *the daughter of famous Arthur and Katherine Murray who taught America to dance,* have dedicated their lives to educating the world about the life-saving Heimlich Maneuver. See: *heimlichinstitute.org*

Heimlich Helps Save Drowning Victims

In more than 90% of drowning cases, the victim's lungs fill with fluid. In this situation, it's imperative that the fluid be expelled quickly - because after four or five minutes the likelihood of brain damage increases. Just getting someone out of the water has not changed their condition – if they still have fluid in their lungs their condition is the same as if they were still under water. In all the studies on drowning since 1933, none showed that mouth-to-mouth resuscitation saved drowning victims without first draining water from their lungs. After all, air cannot get into water-filled lungs!

The Heimlich Maneuver expels water from lungs of drowning victims in six to nine seconds – with two to four Heimlich applications. And unlike CPR, when applied correctly, Heimlich is safe and easily mastered by a person new to the procedure. Option: hold drown victim upside down to drain water out, then apply CPR if needed.

First Aid for Choking, Asthma & Drowning Victims
The Heimlich Maneuver

With the VICTIM STANDING or SITTING

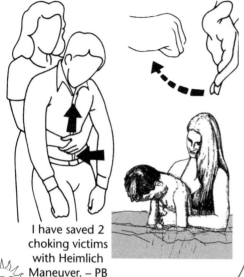

I have saved 2 choking victims with Heimlich Maneuver. – PB

138

1. Stand behind the victim and wrap your arms firmly around their upper waist.

2. Place the thumb side of your fist strongly against the victim's abdomen, slightly just above the navel and below the rib cage.

3. Grasp your fist with your other hand and press fist into upper abdomen with a **quick upward thrust. Repeat often as necessary.**

4. If the victim is sitting, stand behind the victim's chair and perform maneuver in the same manner. Never slap victims' back.

5. **After** food, etc. has been removed, have the victim seen by a doctor immediately.

Note: If you start to choke when alone and help is not available, an attempt should be made to self-administer this Heimlich Maneuver. It works!

When the VICTIM HAS COLLAPSED and CANNOT BE LIFTED:

1. Lay the victim on their back.
2. Face the victim and kneel astride victims hips and thighs.
3. With one hand on top of another, place heel of bottom hand on upper abdomen slightly above navel and below the rib cage.
4. Press into the victim's upper abdomen with a QUICK UPWARD THRUST. Don't squeeze ribcage. Repeat as often as necessary.
5. Should victim vomit, quickly place them on their side and wipe out any vomit from mouth to prevent blocking of throat and aspiration *(drawing vomit into throat). (Ambulances have suction & airway tubes.)*
6. After food, water, etc. is removed, give CPR if needed and it's best to have the victim seen by a doctor immediately.

Everyone should know the versatile Heimlich Maneuver, it's a life-saver!
Check Red Cross classes or Fire Dept. Visit Dr. Heimlich's web: heimlichinstitute.org

Chapter 9

Bathing

The Sixth Step Towards Building Powerful Nerve Force

Cleanliness is next to Godliness. To build powerful Nerve Force we must be clean not only on the inside of our bodies, but on the outside as well. The Bragg Healthy Lifestyle recognizes that a program of eating live, clean and organic foods combined with deep breathing exercises and a fasting program, are all necessary for keeping our bodies healthy, clean and free from toxic poisons.

The body is constantly eliminating toxic poisons through skin pores. Skin is the largest organ of the human body and one of the most important organs of elimination (often called third kidney). Your skin has 96 million pores and they must be kept clean to function properly. Bathing is important not only for cleansing the pores, but is also an aid in building greater Nerve Force. **139**

The toxic poisons come out through the pores of the skin in the form of moisture or water which dries on the skin. This residue must be washed away. That is why it's important to take daily cleansing baths or showers.

We personally think the shower is the best way to cleanse the skin. We like one that has a good pressure. The Wizard Shower Head has the most satisfactory pressure, varying from a fine spray to a forceful spray of water. (Also install filter – see pages 143-145 – on the shower head.)

Your choice of soap is also important. We don't use ordinary commercial soaps, but only pure Castile or a veggie soap with an acid base. You see, it is important not to use alkaline soaps on the body because a healthy skin has an acid base. If you use ordinary soap which is alkaline, you wash away the healthful acid base of the skin. Your skin then gets dry and often becomes irritated. A lot of Nerve Force is lost this way.

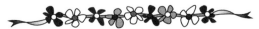

Pure water performs miracles internally and externally for well-being.
– Patricia Bragg, N.D., Ph.D., Pioneering Health Crusader

Cold Water on the Skin is Important For Building Powerful Nerve Force

Cold water – like pure, clean air – is a natural stimulant with no side effects if the body is conditioned to take cold water. After you have washed your body, then you can gradually make the shower colder and colder. After you get conditioned to a cold bath, you will revel in it! Cold water has a great strengthening effect on the nerves.

Also – for even better Nerve Force building – do not use a towel to dry yourself. Use hand massage. Using hand massage on the body while it is wet is a great nerve builder. After your body has been thoroughly dried with your hands, then take a coarse bath towel and give your body a healthy thorough rubbing massage with it.

Cold water, hand rub drying, towel rubbing and skin brushing are tonics to the nerves in the skin. You will tingle with vitality after you make this a part of your daily Bragg Healthy Lifestyle and Exercise Program!

Special Shower Builds Healthy Circulation

Here's a progressive method for improving circulation over your entire body. All you need is a large back brush or Swedish bath friction mitt, Castile soap and a coarse Turkish towel. Now get into shower and turn on hot water. With brush or mitt, gently scrub your body. At first your coddled body won't be able to take too much scrubbing. It's also good to massage neck and upper shoulders. After your scrub/massage, then start to alternate hot and cold showers for 3 to 5 minutes. Now hand, then towel rub dry your body for 3 to 5 minutes – your body circulation will tingle!

Hot/cold water showers are a wonderful way to relax, refresh and stimulate tired muscles. Let the spray beat heavily on your back and shoulders. Occasionally before shower apply Bragg Olive Oil if skin is dry. We advise this relaxing shower before dinner on days when you come home tired. It helps relieve muscular stress and strain!

Start enjoying safe, chlorine-free showers right away. It's essential to ease the strain from your immune system. And you may even get rid of long-standing conditions – from sinus and respiratory problems to dry, itchy skin.

Cold Water Swimmers are Fit and Ageless

My father prides himself on being able to endure the coldest weather wearing only a small amount of clothing, and he has enjoyed swimming in all parts of the world, in all kinds of weather, (which I also enjoy). He is well known for his cold water swimming and is welcomed as a member at *Polar Bear Clubs* worldwide.

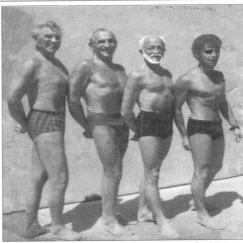

Cold Water Swimmers "L" Street Beach, Boston
Dr. Paul C. Bragg and Dr. John H. Federkiewicz,
David Cooper and Dr. David Carmos (the youngest)

On many occasions, Dad and famous pioneer Dr. Robert Jackson had great sport breaking the ice and swimming with the amazing *Boston Brownies* of the famous "L" Street Bath House in Massachusetts. Here you'll find some of the finest ageless physical specimens in the world, including people in their 60's, 70's, 80's 90's, and even over 100 years.

The same is true of the *Polar Bear*s of Coney Island and at Montrose Beach in Chicago and those at the popular Bradford Beach in Milwaukee, Wisconsin. They are all fit, amazing and ageless. We can truthfully say that all those people who bathed all winter long in the icy waters of the Atlantic Ocean developed the most beautiful skin tone. It really was "the skin you love to touch". One winter Dad and I arrived in New York during a blizzard and found the members of the *Polar Bears* and *Iceberg Club* of Coney Island (both year round bathing clubs) out in full force and we joined them. These robust bathers had absolutely no problem with nervousness and had marvelous skin tone.

Now, we're not advising you to join a year round bather's club, but we are telling you that when the body is conditioned to cold water, there is stronger Nerve Force. That is the reason we want you to condition your body to cold water. It is a great tonic and a natural stimulant.

Check out website: www.polarbearclub.org

Warm and Hot Baths also Have Their Place in Building Nerve Force

There is a time for the cold water bath and there is a time for the warm or hot bath. Say that a person has had a strenuous day during which a great deal of their Nerve Force has been expended and their nerves have been highly keyed up. On this particular day their entire nervous system has been subjected to stress, strain and tension and their nerves feel as if they were tied in knots. This is not the time for the cold water bath! This is definitely a time to take a hot bath – around 102° to 104°F. There is nothing quite as soothing as when you snuggle down into a tub of warm water (add 2 cup vinegar) and let your whole body and nervous system unwind and relax.

We are devotees of both the cold and hot water bath. We had a home in the California Desert near Palm Springs where mineral water comes out of the ground as hot as 167°F. Naturally, you can't bathe in this intense heat, but at the spas we frequent this hot water is cooled down to 104°F. We find it wonderful for our nerves to bathe in this hot mineral water. Not only do these health spas have special soaking pools to enjoy, but they also have swimming pools in which the mineral water is kept at 90°F. In this water swimming is a real tonic for the entire nervous system.

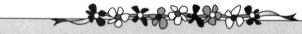

Prayer for Strength & Loving Guidance

I give thanks each day to live a simple, sincere and serene life; repelling promptly every thought of impurity, discontent, anxiety, discouragement and fear. I will continually cultivate health, cheerfulness, happiness, charity and the love of brotherhood; exercising economy in expenditure, generosity in giving, carefulness in conversation and diligence in appointed service. I pledge fidelity to every trust and a childlike faith in God while, in particular, I will be faithful in those habits of prayer, study, work, nutrition, physical exercise, deep breathing and good posture. I shall fast for a 24 hour period each week, eat only natural foods and get sufficient recharging sleep nightly. I will make every effort to improve myself physically, mentally, emotionally and spiritually every day.
– Prayer used by Paul C. Bragg and daughter Patricia Bragg

Five Hidden Dangers in Your Shower:

• **Chlorine:** Added to all municipal water supplies, this disinfectant hardens arteries, destroys proteins in the body, irritates skin and sinus conditions and aggravates any asthma, allergies and respiratory problems.

• **Chloroform:** This powerful by-product of chlorination causes excessive free radical formation (a cause of accelerated ageing!). It causes normal cells to mutate and cholesterol to form. It's a known carcinogen!

• **DCA (Dichloroacetic acid):** This chlorine by-product alters cholesterol metabolism and has been shown to cause liver cancer in lab animals.

• **MX (a chlorinated acid):** Another by-product of chlorination, MX is known to cause genetic mutations that can lead to cancer growth and has been found in all chlorinated water for which it was tested.

• **Proven cause of bladder and rectal cancer:** Research proved that chlorinated water is the direct cause of 9% of all U.S. bladder cancers and 15% of all rectal cancers.

143

Don't Gamble With Your Health – Use a Shower Filter

The most effective method of removing hazards from your shower is the quick and easy installation of a filter on your shower arm. The best filter we found removes chlorine, lead, mercury, iron, chlorine by-products, arsenic, hydrogen sulfide, and many other unseen contaminants, such as bacteria, fungi, dirt and toxic sediments. It has a 12 to 18 month filter life-span and the filter is easily cleaned by backwashing and replaced when needed. I have been using this filter for 3 years and really enjoy my chlorine-free showers! For info on buying best shower filter call weekdays (800) 446-1990.

Start enjoying safe, chlorine-free showers right away. It's essential to reducing your risk of heart disease and cancer and to ease the strain on your immune system. You may even get rid of long-standing conditions – from sinus and respiratory problems, to dry, itchy skin.

We can no more afford to spend major time on minor things, than we can to spend minor time on major things! – Jim Rohn

Showers, Toxic Chemicals & Chlorine

Water chlorination has been widely used to "purify" water in America starting in 1904. But chlorine's negative effects on health surely outweigh any benefits! "Chlorine is the greatest crippler and killer of modern times! While it prevented epidemics of one disease, it was creating another. Twenty years after the start of chlorinating our drinking water, the present mounting epidemic of heart trouble, cancer and senility began in 1924, and is costing billions." – Dr. Joseph Price, *Coronaries, Cholesterol, Chlorine (amazon.com)*

Skin absorption of toxic dangerous contaminants has been greatly underestimated and the ingestion may not constitute the sole primary route of exposure.
– Dr. Halina Brown, *American Journal of Public Health*

Taking long hot showers is a health risk, according to the latest research. Showers – and to a lesser extent baths – lead to a greater exposure to toxic chemicals contained in water supplies than does drinking the water. These toxic chemicals evaporate out of the water and are inhaled. They can also spread through the house and be inhaled by others. People get six to 100 times more chemicals by breathing the air while taking showers and baths than they would by drinking the water. – Ian Anderson, *New Scientist*

144

A Professor of Water Chemistry at the University of Pittsburgh claims that exposure to vaporized chemicals in the water through showering, bathing and inhalation is 100 times greater than through drinking the chemicals in water.
– *The Nader Report – Troubled Waters on Tap*

CHECK FOLLOWING WEBSITES FOR FLUORIDE UPDATES:

- www.voteoutfluoride.com
- www.fluoridealert.org
- www.fluorideresearch.com
- www.bruha.com/fluoride
- www.mercola.com
- www.fluoridation.com
- www.dentalwellness4u.com/oralhealth/fluoride.html
- www.keepers-of-the-well.org

11 Assoc. Stopped Endorsing Water Fluoridation in 1996

- *American Heart Association*
- *American Cancer Society*
- *American Diabetes Association*
- *American Civil Liberties Union*
- *American Chiropractic Association*
- *Society of Toxicology*
- *National Kidney Foundation*
- *American Psychiatric Assoc.*
- *American Academy of Allergy & Immunology*
- *Chronic Fatigue Syndrome Action Network*
- *National Institute of Law Municipal Officers*

You Get More Toxic Exposure from Taking a Chlorinated Water Shower Than From Drinking the Same Water!

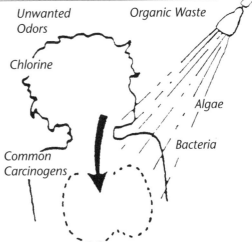

*Two highly volatile and toxic chemicals, are trichloroethylene and toxic chloroform have been proven as contaminants and are in most municipal drinking-water supplies. The great National Academy of Sciences has estimated that 200 to 1,000 people die in the United States each year from the cancers caused largely by ingesting water pollutants from inhalation as air pollutants in the home. Inhalation exposure to water pollutants has largely been ignored. Data indicates that hot showers can liberate about 50% of the chloroform and 80% of the trichloroethylene into air, both toxic chemicals!

Tests show that your body can absorb more toxic chlorine as a result of a 10-minute shower than if you drank 8 glasses of the same water. How can that be?

A warm shower opens up your pores, causing your skin to act like a sponge. As a result, you not only inhale the chlorine vapors, you absorb them through your skin, directly into your bloodstream – at a rate that's up to 6 times higher than if you were directly drinking it. "In terms of the cumulative damage to your health, showering in toxic chlorinated water is one of the most dangerous risks you take daily! Short-term risks include: eyes, sinus, throat, skin and lung irritation. Long-term risks include: excessive free radical formation (that ages you faster!), higher vulnerability to genetic mutation and cancer development; and difficulty in metabolizing cholesterol, causing hardened arteries." *from Science News

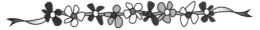

We grow healthier in life with pure water, healthy foods and love!

Swimming is a Great Nerve Force Builder

Swimming is one of the greatest exercises for building Nerve Force. In our lifelong study of athletic sports, we have found that swimmers have the best reserves of Nerve Force. There is something about swimming that has a relaxing effect on the whole nervous system. If either of us were President of the United States, we would have thousands of swimming pools built so that they would be available for everyone! In our opinion, swimming is definitely a great Health and Nerve Builder.

We are writing this book in beautiful Hawaii, where there is some of the finest swimming in the world. We urge you to find a clean safe ocean, river, lake, stream or swimming pool and make swimming a part of your exercise when possible. (Wear ear plugs and eye goggles.) Don't tell us that you are afraid of the water or that you can't swim! It's possible to banish your fears of the water and learn to swim with the help of a competent instructor.

Years ago on the beach at Waikiki we met a woman who was 78 years young. All her life, she had lived with a dread of the water and consequently could not swim. But she came to Hawaii determined to learn how to swim and banish her fears. After a few months she had accomplished both of her goals! She told us that during the greater part of her life she had been a victim of nerves and a poor sleeper. Since she learned to swim, however, her nervousness had completely disappeared and she was now sleeping like a healthy and happy newborn baby!

We urge you to make swimming a part of your life, too. You will find it a non-strenuous sport and a constant source of pleasure – as well as a great Nerve Force builder. Make use of the great health-building power of water!

THE LAW OF CAUSE AND EFFECT

*An unhealthy lifestyle produces illnesses and disease. Most humans are lacking good nutrition and pure water to maintain optimum health! **Fact:** most people are dehydrated. 8 glasses distilled water daily (add 2 tsps Bragg Vinegar to 3) is vital to operate body functions, brain, nerves, energy, etc. and to achieve Powerful Nerve Force for Super Health!*
– Paul C. Bragg, N.D., Ph.D., Life Extension Specialist

Enjoy Energy from Gentle Sunbathing

All living things on earth depend on solar energy for their existence. The sun is the primary source of energy. Earth would be a barren, frigid place if it were not for the magic rays of the sun! All things that live, breathe and grow need the energy of the sun. Sun gives us light, and were it not for light, there would be no you or me. Earth would be in total darkness and void of life. (We endorse solar energy when and where possible.) Mankind can gain health, vitality and happiness in the gentle, healing rays of the sun.

The people who are indoors too long have sallow, ghostly-looking skin. That is why so many women hide their sun-starved skins with face makeup. People who are deprived of the vital rays of the sun have a half-dead look. They are actually dying for want of solar energy! The direct rays of the gentle sun on the naked body supply vitality and dynamic energy and recharge the human storage battery with renewed strength to build powerful and vibrant Nerve Force! Life-giving sunshine is essential to your health, happiness and longevity.

147

The rays of the sun are powerful germicides. As the skin imbibes more of these rays, it stores up enormous amounts of this germ-killing energy. The gentle sun provides a remedy for the nervous person filled with anxiety, worry, stresses and strains. When these tense people lie in the early morning or late afternoon gentle sunshine, its healing rays give them what the nerves and body are crying out for . . . and that is relaxation!

Vitamin D3 is made when UVB light from the sun is absorbed by the skin. This is the most natural form. Most supplements sold today are Vitamin D3 (animal source – lanolin) or Vitamin D2 (fungus/yeast derived) ideal for vegetarians/vegans. Vitamin D3 is more potent form of Vitamin D and has a better stable shelf-life. Learn more by reading "Vitamin D Solution" by Michael F. Holick, Ph.D., M.D., Professor Boston University and recipient of prestigious "Linus Pauling Prize" for his extensive research on Vitamin D.

Daily intakes of Vitamin D of (at least) 4,000 IU are needed to reduce the risk of cancers, Multiple Sclerosis and Type 1 Diabetes. Only about 10% of the U.S. population has levels in this range, mainly people who work outdoors. Sunlight is a prime source of Vitamin D. Fish oil and soymilk are two excellent sources of Vitamin D. Check with your health care practitioner or nutritionist to determine your optimum Vitamin D intake.

Gentle Sunbathing Works Miracles!

When you begin sunbathing, start with short time periods until you condition your body to take more. The best time for beginners to start taking 10 and 15 minute sunbaths is in the early morning sunshine until 10 a.m. or late afternoon sunshine after 3 p.m. Between 11 and 3 we usually avoid stronger, burning rays. Please don't use sunscreen, the chemicals are harmful. Sunscreens do not prevent skin cancers, they promote them. When absorbed through the skin, they disrupt our body's balanced hormone ecosystem (we wear straw hats). Read Elizabeth Plourde's new book, *Sunscreens – Biohazard: Treat as Hazardous Waste* (*amazon.com*). See web: *www.sunscreensbiohazard.com*.

The cool rays of the sun rejuvenate the skin and help keep our eyes healthy and in focus. The gentle sun is a tonic for frazzled nerves. Its cool rays calm, quiet and soothe the nerves while helping to promote a relaxed feeling. You can combine a nap with a sunbath, you will help refill the body reservoirs with Nerve Force. After gently sunning, pat on some Bragg Apple Cider Vinegar.

148

Enjoy God's Sunshine for Super Health

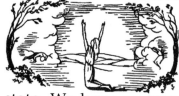 That is why my father and I have always loved God's own precious sunshine. That's why we made our main home in California, the great sunshine state. We have an organic farm in Santa Barbara near the ocean where we get the benefits of the clean air and sunshine. We also live part-time in Hawaii so we can visit with the Bragg readers who visit our free Bragg Exercise Class (see page iii) at famous Waikiki Beach. The class is 6 days a week and it's fun to exercise in the fresh clean ocean air. We enjoy our students who come from all over the world. Seek fresh, clean air, gentle sunshine and organic sun-kissed foods, then soon super health will leap out and be yours to treasure throughout a long, ever youthful, productive, happy life!

Gentle sunshine is a soothing tonic, a stimulant and a Great Healer for the body, also sunshine is healthy for eyes! As you bask in the warm, gentle sunshine (not hot afternoon sun), millions of nerve endings absorb the energy from the sun and transform it so the body's nervous system can use it.

Chapter 10

Keep Your Emotions Under Control

The Seventh Step to Building A Powerful Nerve Force

Common sense dictates that one of the first steps toward greater Nerve Force consists in checking the waste of Nerve Force squandered in unnecessary emotions. When you have learned to expend less Nerve Force than your nervous system develops, this brings you more real peace and power mentally, physically, emotionally and spiritually.

Follow These Stress Reducing Guidelines:

Avoid the super-person complex! Some people want too much from themselves. They are perfectionists. They are full of tensions from pushing themselves **149** beyond their human capacity to perform. We believe in perfection, but not at the cost of nerve exhaustion! One person cannot be skilled in everything. Do your best with those tasks which you cannot do so well and let it go at that. No one asks or expects you to accomplish the impossible, so don't demand it of yourself! You will have a much longer, healthier and happier life.

Talk out your worries! Don't bottle everything up. If you feel you have a legitimate "beef" against someone, go to that person and quietly talk things out. Just as it takes a good storm to clear up the atmosphere when the weather is "tense", a good talk will usually clear up a disturbed emotional atmosphere. Do not harbor resentments! Get them off your chest quickly and calmly as possible! Nine times out of ten they arise from a misunderstanding – either on your part, the other person's or both.

Whatever occurs in the mind, effects the body and visa versa. Mind and body cannot be considered independently. When the two are out of sync, both the emotional and physical stress can erupt.
– Hippocrates, the Father of Medicine, 400 B.C.

This applies to all relationships – whether it be your mate, children, in-laws, relatives, friends or your co-workers, etc. So many husbands and wives or parents and children have let resentments build up inside until they can no longer communicate with one another. They have built a wall out of pebbles! If you have let things get to this stage, you might be heading for a nervous breakdown! You may need to place your confidence in a good friend, therapist, relative or clergyman. Talking things over with someone who can be objective will relieve stress and enable you to view your plight in a clear light and help you find a logical solution to your worry or problem.

Beware of your temper. Temper is too good a thing to lose! Under control, your temper becomes a driving force that can push you forward to the accomplishment of worthwhile goals. Out of control, your temper can destroy you, your relationships, business and others as well.

When you get irate you are wasting your Nerve Force. You are throwing away precious nerve energy. A "fit of temper" often causes nervous and physical exhaustion.

Start counting and keep on counting when you feel your temper rising. Don't say anything you will regret! Get into some vigorous physical activity at once. The best way to cool your anger is to take a brisk walk in the open air. Get away from the person or situation that is sending you into a rage. No matter how good you might feel after you "tell them off" you will lose precious Nerve Force in doing so. Swimming, gardening, housework or any other type of physical work or exercise will help work off your temper and use that Nerve Force constructively.

Don't resort to physical violence when your temper rises. The answer is not in fighting, hitting or beating! That is how crimes and murders are committed! Channel and exercise that unleashed nerve energy into constructive activities that will harm no one – yourself or anyone else. Keep your temper under healthy control at all times!

A Harvard Study shows that men with highest anger on personality tests are three times more likely to develop heart disease. High blood pressure affects 1 in 3 of all adults in the U.S.; it is often called "the silent killer".

In the Framingham Heart Study, women who reported suppressing their anger experienced the highest rate of first heart attacks.

Avoid Arguing, Teasing & Nagging

Thousands of murders have been committed and endless hatred, bitterness and anger have resulted from heated arguments that had their beginnings in a friendly discussion of a trivial subject. An argument is a form of mental combat. We fully realize that discussions and arguments can sharpen one's wits and are often highly instructive. There are few people, however, who can indulge in a friendly argument without becoming unduly excited. Such excitement is one of the greatest forms of nerve strain and should be avoided by people who must conserve their Nerve Force. We have met with hundreds of people suffering from nerve disorders which were due mainly to this negative habit of nerve abuse.

The worst time in the world to get into any kind of argument is at mealtime. If there is anything that will completely upset your digestion, it's arguing when you are eating! We both believe that constant arguments at the table can bring on ulcers and indigestion.

151

When a person with sensitive nerves – who is likely to become unduly excited – realizes that a discussion has reached a combative stage, that particular conversation should be discontinued at once. A good plan is to state simply, "You may be right. At least I shall not argue the matter further with you at this present time."

Don't quarrel. Don't nag or tease and do not permit yourself to be nagged or teased. Avoid people who do so. If you allow someone to "get your goat" they will be tempted to continue plaguing you. But if you appear impervious, ignore them or simply walk away in silence they're likely to let you alone.

There are personalities that just do not mix well. Not everyone whom you come in contact with is going to like you or agree with your ideas! The same holds true from your point of view. Learn to live and let live! In our busy lives we've come into contact with people who irritate us. We keep out of their way, avoid them! Even with family there will be some who irritate you. Just keep your distance from them.

Before speaking – put it to the test: Is it good? Is it kind? Is it necessary?

Don't argue with them – it burns up precious Nerve Force! Don't try to convert them to your ideas or philosophy unless willing – then share a Bragg book with them or one suggested on page 70.

Don't hate these people. When you hate a person you are destroying yourself! Look upon these people as you would a bad odor – simply stay away from them! If you're forced to be in their company be pleasant but have as little to say to them as possible.

Shun Constant Suspicion

Many people make themselves unhappy, poison their minds and strain their nerves with extreme suspicion. They are constantly living in fear that someone is trying to cheat, rob or deceive them. They believe in the doctrine that "Everyone is a thief until proven otherwise."

This extreme suspicion may save a person a few dollars during their lifetime and may occasionally prevent them from being deceived . . . but does it pay? Is it fair toward those who are honest? We don't think so – because it wrecks one's health! Granted, you may be cheated occasionally, but we consider such money better lost than spent on nerve drugs and doctors!

Reap the Rewards of Smiling

Here's a great old wise saying, **"Laugh and the world laughs with you. Cry and you cry alone."** It has often been truly stated that the act of laughing causes certain beneficial vibrations that promote circulation in the vital abdominal region. We are also thoroughly convinced that laughing promotes health because this positive mental condition prompts laughter (see page 153). Make an angry face, soon you will feel grouchy and ready to resent the slightest offense – real or fancied. This negative mental attitude depresses the nerves, and effects the heart and lungs and so on. Laughing produces the opposite – a positive effect upon your entire being! Read the classic, *Anatomy of an Illness* by Norman Cousins. This famous book reinforces these principles! Seek out happy, humorous books and videos. Also choose radio and TV programs that make you laugh and smile!

Cheerfulness is the atmosphere under which all things thrive. – Richter

Happy Feelings Are Internal Smiles

Try this experiment. Stop reading and smile. Do you feel unaccountably happy internally, although at the moment you may not have a special reason to be happy? Now make an angry face. You will observe that you feel angry. If we placed a sphygmograph on your wrist to record your heart pulsations and blood waves, the tracings would show a decided depression in your heart action, proving that your forced grouchy attitude has caused an immediate depression of all your vital organs. So practice smiling! Smile when you read, when you are tranquil and while at rest. Smile when you are angry or worried. Eventually the smile will grow on your face and give you a happy expression. That external smile will soon give you a happy feeling inside – an internal smile!

Keep away from people who have those dark and gloomy expressions on their faces. That is one reason we like to be with young children and healthy teenagers. They laugh. There does not have to be too much to laugh at to produce their warm, natural laughter. We also like to be around people who have a good sense of humor. We love people who keep young at heart, kind and considerate, regardless of their calendar years? Emotions are contagious. Be around people who feel happy and you will feel happy too! Smile and almost always you will get a smile in response.

Instant Mood Lifters

If you're feeling a little blue, don't give yourself some phony pep talk! Have handy a list of positive actions you can take that will lift your spirits! After all, actions always speak louder – and do more – than words.

Here are Some Tried & True Mood Builders:

Take a brisk walk. Exercise outdoors in fresh air and sunshine, it always has positive effects on your total health.

Spend time with a young child. Their simple outlook on life is a reminder that things aren't as bad as you think. Being childlike at times has merit! Enjoy your pets.

Share smiles – we shall never know all the good a simple smile can do!

Those who bring sunshine to the lives of others cannot keep it from themselves. – James Matthew Barrie, Peter Pan Creator

Laughter does miracles! Read the cartoon (funny) pages. Childlike simplicity is refreshing. Learn to find the absurdly humor in whatever is bothering you. As someone once said, "Don't take life so seriously, because you never get out of it alive anyway."

Take a moment to walk in the other persons shoes. If someone has upset you, think about the problems and sorrows in their life. This allows for some perspective on the situation and maybe some solutions.

Pretend you're happy. It sounds silly, but it works! If you smile and act happy, your body responds similarly. In many instances, being happy or content is a matter of choice. American sociologist M. Kathleen Casey says, "Pain is inevitable, suffering is optional." Much of our emotional and physical suffering can be alleviated by mind-body techniques because they are intertwined and want to heal each other. These techniques can help neutralize stress and even pain on our bodies.

154 Remove Negative Chips Off Your Shoulders

Don't be too sensitive! If a person says a cutting thing to you, forget it! Don't make a big issue of it and waste your vital Nerve Force arguing about it. Most mean people are usually unhealthy and mentally sick. Don't stoop down to their low level! Brush them off as you would a fly. Life is too precious to let others pull you down – and they can't unless you allow it! Many mentally sick people do try to get others down because "misery loves company". Don't join them! Avoid them!

Let the other fellow hate, envy, be jealous and live a negative mental life. Not you! Be too smart to let this kind of thinking sicken you. In our long lives, we have known people who actually poisoned themselves to death with their violent hatreds! Uncontrolled emotions can make you sick, unhappy nervous and a physical wreck.

For heaven's sake, please stop looking for perfection in people! We all have some weaknesses and there are no 100% perfect humans. Try to see the good in people you are thrown in contact with and also in yourself!

Nothing transforms a person as much as changing from a negative attitude to a healthy positive attitude.

Paul Bragg Practiced Thought Substitution

My father's mother was a wise and noble woman who had a splendid philosophy to guide us. It was she who taught Dad thought substitution. He remembers it well:

"My constant companion was a little dog named Wilbur, whom I loved very dearly. One day Wilbur was killed. Heartbroken, I came to my mother with my grief. As I sobbed in her arms, she told me how to conquer the pain of my loss with thought substitution. Instead of grieving over my dog, she told me that I should change my thoughts to the happy times I had with Wilbur – such as the long hikes in the springtime when the dogwood was in bloom, or the way Wilbur used to scare a rabbit and give chase, but the rabbit would always outsmart Wilbur. Before I realized it, I was laughing through my tears as I recalled my good times with Wilbur. From then on, whenever I would think about my dog, I would automatically replace my sense of loss with a happy memory."

"Through my mother's guidance I learned to apply healthy *thought substitution (visualization) when needed to other sorrows. The substitution of happy thoughts for sad ones saved my emotional Nerve Force throughout my life! Grief over the loss of a loved one is the greatest of all nerve strains. It may depress the nervous system enough to cause death. I know such grief. In spite of my positive philosophy and my remarkable physical stamina, I have lost many pounds in just days through intense grief and found my vital organs, especially my heart and lungs, so depressed that I found it difficult to breathe. I know how hard it is to bring grief under control, but it can be done! Thought substitution is the secret."*

Only one thought can occupy the mind at any one time. By an effort of will we can force out the grief-stricken, unhappy thoughts and replace them with tender, happy memories. Sorrow is a futile waste of Nerve Force. Tears cannot erase the cause of grief or emotional torment of any kind. This useless waste of nerve energy can be stopped with thought substitution (visualization). Let happy, positive thoughts occupy your mind. It all comes back to the saying ***The kingdom of heaven is within you. It's within your power to make your kingdom a wonderful, inspiring, relaxing, stress-free heaven on earth!***

Don't Batter Yourself with Self-Torture

Combat grief and other emotional plagues by keeping your mind free from the depressing subject. Divert your inner thoughts into other constructive directions. Most important of all, do not form the morbid habit of finding perverse pleasure in the torture of grief or other emotional pain! We have carefully studied persons who were victims of intense grief or hurt and in nearly every instance we found that they purposefully tortured themselves – just as some fanatical religious sects find masochistic pleasure in self-inflicted pain from fire, lashings, snake bites and other means of self-abuse.

This form of insanity should not be encouraged by giving such persons our sympathy since this only makes matters worse. Do not encourage those who wallow in grief by offering them your sympathy! Talk uplifting, positive common sense to them. If you are the victim of deep depression, grief or other emotional pain, remember you and you alone must overcome your grief or pain! Thought substitution and clear, unemotional thinking are your strong weapons. Life is a vale of tears. Unfortunately some grief and sorrow are parts of life that we must learn to adjust to. We must learn to control our emotions, not let our emotions control us!

Send Your Worry to the Winds

As we stated earlier in this book, worry can destroy you if you let it get the upper hand. Worry – like grief – is greatly exaggerated by many people and is employed as a means of self-torture. Many people enlarge their worries so that they may be pitied and petted – a selfish practice.

It's true worry is often unavoidable, like war, etc. We can't always turn our backs upon it, especially if it means business ruin, loss of love, poverty, etc. But we can always use clear thinking, common sense and good judgment to our advantage! We should bar worry from our minds since we know little can be gained by it.

Having a bad day? Try walking around the block several times or run up and down a few flights of stairs. You'll return to the task at hand less troubled because the physiological changes caused by even moderate exercise calms the mind.

On the contrary, the more we worry, the greater the strain on our Nerve Force and the less able we'll be to overcome our troubles. We should remain optimistic in the face of all obstacles! Remember it is always the positive optimist who succeeds, never the negative pessimist.

Millions of people worry endlessly about trivial matters, making mountains out of molehills. Many of these worries arise from excessive vanity, false pride, egotism and conceit. For example, people worry when they see their first few gray hairs on their head and let themselves get brainwashed by the peddlers of hair dye. Some people constantly worry about what other people may think of them or say about them. Women especially seem to be victims of those petty concerns which undermine their health and prematurely wrinkle their faces, while they sour their minds and dispositions.

Children – and especially teenagers – are the cause of much worry today. Teenagers are the victims of herd psychology and sincerely believe that they must do whatever the others in their group are doing. If you **157** have teenagers, it is your duty to teach them to think for themselves! They must learn that just because the herd does a stupid, bad or silly thing, that is no reason why everyone should be silly or stupid. Most adults cannot communicate with their teenage children. You must find a way to talk with them if you are going to help them through this rough period of their lives. It is a very tough and cruel world that teenagers face today. You must give them all the guidance possible to start them in the right direction towards the good life. Worrying and wringing your hands won't do it! Send worries to the winds and let good health and clear thinking refresh your mind.

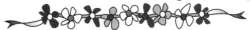

Any time you get upset it tears down your nervous system. – Mae West

Living in harmony with the universe is living totally alive, full of vitality, health, joy, inner peace, power, love, and abundance on every level. – Shakti Gawain

Things which matter most should never be at the mercy of things which matter least. – Goethe

Remember what really matters in life – is what you do with what you have – your talents, gifts, knowledge, strengths, beliefs, etc.!

Become a Practical Healthy Idealist

We'd like to state here that we consider the advice and teachings of most "idealists" and psychologists as very impractical. We do not believe that all psychological problems can be solved on the mental level. We believe that a lot of our mental problems are caused by an unhealthy lifestyle! If you eat foods deficient in B-Complex vitamins and calcium, all the psychological treatments in the world are not going to put these important nerve nutrients into your body. Nor are they going to clean the toxic poisons out of your body and allow more oxygen to flow into your nervous system.

Human beings are composed of mind, body and spirit, but we must recognize the weakness of our body first because it is often the cause of mental and physical ill health. We firmly believe in meditation and prayer, but unless there is a program of physical fitness and diet along with it, it's almost worthless! We believe bliss consciousness comes when we work on the physical, mental and spiritual planes! Some idealists tell us that disease and pain do not exist, that we should rise so high in our mental poise that we are above worry, grief or anger and that evil ceases to exist – NOT TRUE! We are as idealistic as any of these dreamers, but we are practical idealists who keep our feet on firm earth and do not permit false theories to carry us away.

The health teachings we've set forth here are basic and thoroughly practical! They do not suggest or rely upon the impossible. With effort you can protect your nerves from undue torture and strain while you make giant strides toward building greater Nerve Force and health.

A Strong Mind in a Strong Body

To be able to live in a world of diversity and differing opinions, you have self-control, with a strong mind in a strong body. These will always be in balance if you follow our program for building powerful Nerve Force. You can enjoy the highest health state of human existence – Bliss Consciousness – a peace of mind, body and spirit over-flowing with serenity, happiness and joy of living!

The great thing in life is not so much where you stand,
but in what direction you are moving, either healthy or unhealthy.

Chapter 11

Healthy Relaxation: How to Relax the Nerves

The Eighth Step to Building A Powerful Nerve Force

The word "relax" is very much like the word "love." When you ask the average person what it means to relax, you get all kinds of different answers – just as you do when you ask for a definition of love.

We often hear people say at our athletic club, "I want to smoke a cigarette and relax." For others it's whiskey and soda, a cup of coffee, tea or an ice cold cola. None of these people have the slightest idea what the word relax means! They are all talking about stimulants! It is impossible to relax when you are pouring alcohol, tobacco, coffee, tea and cola drinks into your system. This is the opposite of relaxing. This is whipping your nerves with powerful drug stimulants.

Let's get the correct definition of the word relax and then we will carry on from there. Webster's dictionary says, *Relax: to make less tense or rigid; to become less intense or severe; to cast off social restraint, nervous tension or anxiety; to seek rest or recreation.* We think these definitions are the correct meaning of the word relax. You cannot relax in the true sense of the word when you use stimulants and powerful drugs. We'll admit that stimulants and drugs will deaden the nerves for a time. You can give a person a powerful sedative and it will temporarily calm them, or – in many cases – knock a person out cold. Some sedatives will put a person into a deep stupor, but it is impossible to say that these people are relaxed – they are drugged!

Caffeine: *Increases blood pressure, depletes calcium and magnesium from body, elevates cholesterol levels and increases level of dangerous homocysteine in blood. When your coffee high wears off, you feel the drop in terms of fatigue, irritability, headache and confusion.*
– *Caffeine Blues* by Stephen Cherniske, M.S. (amazon.com)

159

People use the word relax very carelessly. Some will tell you they are going on a trip to relax and get away from all the tensions of their lives. While this may help relieve daily stress, bad habits of living are carried along. We will admit that a trip can refresh you – but true relaxation comes from removing bad lifestyle habits.

Relaxation is a Healthy, Soothing Feeling

Relaxation is a special feeling. There is no other way to express it. This feeling is not something you can turn off and on at will. It is something that must be built up in the conscious and the subconscious mind, something you build up in every one of the billions of cells in your body, in your entire nervous system, in your vital organs and in your muscles.

There have been times – yes, many times – when you have correctly let your feelings direct your life. Haven't you said to yourself more than once, "I have a feeling I should not go on that trip as I planned to do?" Let's say it was to be a plane trip. So you listened to the inner voice of your feelings and did not go. Then something came up in your life that made you glad you didn't go. You relied upon your feelings.

We have often said, "I have a feeling that person doesn't like me." Sure enough, we find that person trying to undermine our character to others. Or, someone hurts you dreadfully and you say to them, "You have hurt my feelings." You feel the hurt deep inside.

Yes, we do have feelings and we do feel things. Relaxation is a feeling. Your feelings allow your nerves to relax. Your feelings can banish stress, strain and tensions to bring calm, inner peace and serenity. Feeling is the life force within you that is always working for you. All it needs is a chance. It is astonishing how few people get their physical, mental and emotional debris out of the way and let feeling work for them.

The greatest discovery of my generation is that human beings can alter their lives by altering their attitudes of mind. – William James (1842-1920)

Where your focus goes – your energy flows.

In times of stress be bold, strong and valiant. – Horace, 65 B.C.

Everyone knows what it is to feel *miserable* . . . just as everyone knows how it feels to be tired, exhausted, weak, sad or depressed. All people know what pain feels like. Our feelings do not deceive us. We all know how we feel when we get up in the morning. We know how we feel during the day. Feeling is a vital part of our lives!

If we feel nervous, weak, tired and miserable we produced those feelings with our incorrect daily living habits. Feeling follows the law of cause and effect. Every effect in life is produced by a cause. You get out of life just what you put into it. It is one of the great and inflexible laws of life. Most people are plagued with stress, strains and tensions. These conditions do not just appear out of a blue sky! They are motivated by a cause.

Relaxation is a feeling produced by one's actions, attitude and environment. If you follow a defined program of building Nerve Force, you can produce the feeling of complete relaxation! However, you must earn this feeling. There is no use trying to get it with a cigarette, cup of coffee, tea, cola or an alcoholic drink. **161**

Tension and Relaxation Create the Heartbeat of Life

As you obey and live by the Laws of Mother Nature you'll automatically earn the right to relax when your body needs relaxation. There is nothing wrong with tension. Tension is part of life. For example – when we walk out onto the platform to lecture before 5,000 people for 2 hours we are bound to feel some tension! Life is movement and movement requires tension as well as release. How is that fact expressed in your body?

You have a miraculous muscle in your chest cavity that is active from the moment it begins to function before birth to the instant of your death. That miracle muscle is your heart. How does it keep going for so many years? Study it closely. Observe exactly how it works. It tenses and then relaxes, tenses and relaxes. Thus it can go on and on and on. There is a great lesson for us here.

Open your mind for the doors of wisdom are never shut! – Ben Franklin

Be kind to your heart – it takes care of you and keeps you alive!!!

The heart is like life itself. It should be made up of tension and relaxation. To get a task done – whether it is large or small – we must draw upon our Nerve Force reserves. We put an extra push into our efforts and this extra push is tension. If our nerves are healthy and we are working correctly, when the effort of the task is over we should automatically have the feeling of relaxation.

You can't force relaxation any more than you can change the beating of your heart. Relaxation is a feeling, always remember that. It is something that works naturally within your nervous system. Live by Mother Nature's Laws and you will never have to worry about relaxation. This feeling will come to you naturally.

Pay no attention to people who tell you to relax, unless they also tell you how to tense for action and how to coordinate the two states. Life is ebb and flow. It is part of life to tense when necessary – and then to relax. We have heard lecturers tell students to "let go"– to lie in bed and raise a leg, then drop it and tell the leg it is completely relaxed. Do the same with an arm. These are good exercises, but true relaxation takes more than exercise. Relaxation is a beautiful soothing feeling within your body and mind.

Strive to make your nervous system so powerful that your body will automatically shift from tension to relaxation. This will be your natural rhythm of living if you earn it by healthful living. It is the great law of compensation at work. Under the wise Laws of Mother Nature you only get what you earn. There is a price tag for everything in life. You get absolutely nothing for nothing. You must earn the feeling of true relaxation. You cannot get it with artificial chemicals.

Be good to your body and it will be good to you! Abuse the body and it will punish you with tension, stress, strain, even constipation! The Laws of Mother Nature don't punish you – you punish yourself! Live so that the feeling of relaxation will come to you when it is needed. Be a friend to yourself! Treat yourself right so you can enjoy a long, healthy and relaxed life. *The kingdom of heaven is within.* When your body is completely relaxed then you will experience an inner peace, inner serenity and the true joy of living.

Healthy remedies such as warm baths, saunas, steam rooms and long walks in nature go a long way in improving your overall health.

There are No Magic Cures

No drug exists that will build Nerve Force. All artificial stimulants such as coffee, tea, tobacco, colas, alcohol and drugs are in a low rate of vibration. These will dissipate, drain and damage your Nerve Force, not build it. Yes, there are drugs that will push or quiet your nerves such as pep pills, etc. which so many nervous cripples use daily to keep them going. There are drugs that will stun and quiet the nerves when they are unmanageable. But no conscientious health practitioner will prescribe these drugs except when absolutely necessary to tide a patient over a crisis.

There are no magic, quick cures for people who have exhausted their Nerve Force that will build Nerve Force or "tone up" the body and its many functions. Nutritional supplements, herbs, etc. and Chiropractic, massage, exercise, special baths, etc., are all valuable therapies, but only as local treatments. Only you can strike at the root of nerve or functional weaknesses by your lifestyle – how you live and the way you think!

There is only one sure way to have powerful Nerve Force . . . you must build it by adopting a constructive program of living. We wish there were shortcuts that we could recommend to you. We are all controlled by the law of compensation. You get nothing for nothing. To build powerful Nerve Force, you must work at it each day of your life. It is through knowledge and wisdom that we achieve the good things in life. It is through positive thinking and positive action that we build supreme, awesome vitality and super Nerve Force. Start now!

Ten Little, Two-Letter Words of Action To Say Daily:

If it is to be, it is up to me!

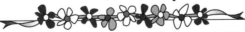

Free yourself from bondage of these killing habits:

- ❤ "I will not use tobacco."
- ❤ "I will not over-eat."
- ❤ "I will not drink black tea."
- ❤ "I will not use salt."
- ❤ "I will not drink coffee, sodas and alcoholic drinks."
- ❤ "I will not clog my arteries with saturated fats."

Be your own health captain and do what needs to be done for your health!

Ten Great No-Calorie Stress Busters:

1. Turn on your favorite music and dance.
2. Enroll in a yoga class, or take tai chi, chi gong, Pilates or stretching class.
3. Call a good friend and have some laughs.
4. Read inspiring Bragg books and health magazines.
5. Take a hot herbal bubble bath or vinegar bath.
6. Go to the gym or take a brisk fresh air walk.
7. Get a massage – best at home when possible.
8. Write and release your feelings in daily journal.
9. Watch an inspiring movie, comedy or travelogue.
10. Close your eyes, relax, do 'yoga breathing' – breathe in slowly through nose, letting air fill lungs completely down to the diaphragm. Hold in briefly, then exhale through the mouth slowly. See: *healthandyoga.com.*

164

The Benefits of Full Yoga Breathing

- Helps release acute and chronic muscular tensions in the body, especially around the heart and digestive organs.
- Increases lung capacity – this helps asthma and emphysema sufferers overcome fear of having shortness of breath attacks.
- Encourages proper nervous stimulus to the cardiovascular system.
- Dramatically reduces emotional and nervous anxiety.
- Helps detox by increasing carbon dioxide and oxygen exchange.
- Helps auto-immune system by increased energy to endocrine system that regulates metabolism, tissue function, internal temperature, water balance, ions and your personality moods.
- Calms the mind and integrates the mental and physical balance.
- Contributes to vitality, energy and relaxation.

As often as possible make yourself smile and laugh; it opens the blood vessels in the back of your head to physically lift your mood. Choose to be happy in spite of circumstances. You can make yourself happy, it's your inner Nerve Force and attitude that sparkles from within.

Dancing Helps Your Heart: *A recent study has found that dancing has the same benefit for heart patients as working out at the gym. Hit the dance floor and help your heart said* readersdigest.com. I love dancing! I've danced the Polka on TV show with Lawrence Welk. I danced with Fred Astaire, Gene Kelly, Bob Hope and Arthur Murray said, *"You dance like a feather, you're the same size as my wife Katherine."* See: *bragg.com/blog/?s=MURRAY* for a fun Arthur Murray teaching video. – PB

Chapter 12

Enjoy Life!

The Ninth Step to Building A Powerful Nerve Force

Learn to Live Joyously with Yourself

Remember you came into this world alone and leave it alone. It's nice to have a good family, friends and a mate, but – above all – you must learn to love living with yourself! Don't become too intimate with too many people because "familiarity often breeds contempt". Maintain a high personal dignity level, even with yourself. You must be good company for yourself. We have never been bored in our lives. We go on long hikes and get to understand ourselves better. As we grow to understand ourselves better, we get to understand other humans more.

165

Lead a busy, happy, creative life. If you follow our Nerve Force Building Program, you are going to be busy! You will have a happy, well-rounded, balanced day with your meditation and prayer, your exercises and deep breathing, healthy eating program and reading new, instructive books, plus continuing with your daily work. A busy person is a happy person with little time to worry. Life becomes a great adventure. Enjoy every minute of it! We only get 24 precious hours a day. No one gets more – be they king, queen or billionaire. So live each day as though it were your last! Make every minute count! Time is too precious to waste! When someone says, "I have to kill time, I'm bored," we think, "How sad!" Now, accept new challenges. Don't be afraid to tackle any job or chore, no matter how big! Get going and start living healthy and successfully now!

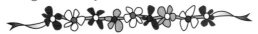

Love, kindness and compassion are necessities, not luxuries without them humanity cannot survive. – The Dalai Lama, a Bragg Follower

The learning process is never ending, and growth will continue, if only you will allow it to. – Arlene Francis

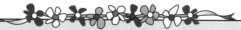

Enjoy Healthy Happy Productive Time

READ THIS POEM OFTEN:
I have just a tiny little minute,
Only sixty seconds in it,
Give account if I abuse it;
Forced upon me; can't refuse it.
Didn't seek it, didn't choose it,
But it's up to me to use it.
Once used – it's gone!
I must suffer if I misuse it . . .
    Use each minute wisely – eternity is in it.

Make Your Own Sunshine & Happiness

166

    Some people's cheerfulness and joy is governed by the weather. When the sun shines brightly, they are bright. When the weather is gloomy, they're gloomy. There are more suicides in gloomy weather than when it's sunny!

    Try the smiling cure. Learn to love the rain when it rains, love darkness when it is dark and love the blazing heat when it is blazing hot. **James Whitcomb Riley wrote:**

> *It is not any use to grumble and complain;*
> *It's just as cheap and easy to rejoice;*
> *When God sorts out the weather and sends rain,*
> *Then, rain's my choice.*

    Singing in the Rain is one of our favorite songs. When you are healthy and happy the weather doesn't bother you. Your disposition is not governed by the barometer. You can make your own sunshine within yourself!!!

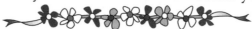

A good laugh is like sunshine in a house. – William Makepeace Thackeray

---

Wherever you go, no matter what the weather,
always bring your own sunshine. – Anthony J. D'Angelo

This is the day which the Lord hath made; we will rejoice and be glad in it.
– Psalms 118:24

Little acts of kindness throughout the day will make your life so much better and bring a little sunshine to others along the way.

My pleasant thoughts bring me peace. – Paul Bragg, N.D., Ph.D.

Have an Attitude of Gratitude!

Gratitude creates happiness because it makes us feel full and complete. Gratitude is the realization that we have everything we need. One of the truths about gratitude is that it is impossible to feel both the positive emotion of thankfulness and a negative emotion such as anger or fear at the same time. Gratitude gives only positive feelings – love, compassion, joy, and hope. As we focus on what we are thankful for, fear, anger, and bitterness simply melt away.*

Enjoy Life – Slow Down

Life has lots of simple things to enjoy. But if you move too fast, you might overlook them. Don't be in such a hurry. Look at the world around you. Notice the grass, the flowers, the sunrise or sunset – Mother Nature is all around you. Take time to pause and reflect.

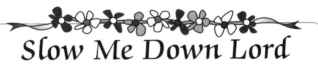

Slow Me Down Lord

Slow me down Lord and fill me with your love.

Ease the pounding of my heart by the quieting of my mind.

Quiet my hurried pace with a vision of eternal time.

Give me, amid the confusion of the day,
the calmness of the everlasting hills.

Break the tensions of my nerves and muscles with the soothing
music of the singing streams that live in my memory.

Help me to know the magical, restoring power of sound sleep.

Teach me the art of taking minute vacations or slowing down
to look at a flower, to chat with a friend, to pat a dog,
to read a few lines from a good book.

Slow me down Lord and inspire me to send my roots deep
into the soil of life's enduring values, so that I may
grow toward the stars of my greater destiny.

An attitude of gratitude creates blessings. – Sir John Templeton

*Excerpt from *Attitudes of Gratitude* by M.J. Ryan

20 Simple Tips to Enjoy Life More

1. Be positive
2. Be generous
3. Enjoy your meal
4. Find a hobby
5. Sing
6. Stay healthy
7. Learn new things
8. Take a walk in the park
9. Gather with friends
10. Find what you love and do it!
11. Go hiking
12. Read a book
13. Share with others
14. Watch a good movie
15. Watch the sunrise
16. Get a massage
17. Be confident
18. Don't worry
19. Spend time with loved ones
20. Relax, give yourself a day off

WE THANK THEE

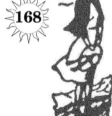

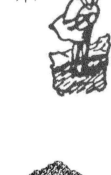

For flowers that bloom about our feet;
For song of bird and hum of bee;
For all things fair we hear or see,
Father in heaven we thank Thee!
For blue of stream and blue of sky;
For pleasant shade of branches high;
For fragrant air and cooling breeze;
For beauty of the blooming trees,
Father in heaven we thank Thee!
For mother love and father care,
For brothers strong and sisters fair;
For love at home and here each day;
For guidance lest we go astray,
Father in heaven we thank Thee!
For this new morning with its light;
For rest and shelter of the night;
For health and food, for love and friends;
For every thing His goodness sends,
Father in heaven we thank Thee!

– Ralph Waldo Emerson

168

Seek first the kingdom of God and all things shall come to you. – Matthew 6:33

Chapter 13

The Biochemistry of Mental Health

Having spent our long lifetimes in the research and practical application of the biochemical relationship between nutrition and human health – and for much of that time having felt like "a voice in the wilderness" – we are happy to have lived long enough to see our Bragg teachings being verified by medical research. For years we have warned people around the world that the increased devitalization and "embalming" of foodstuffs consumed by the general public would result in an alarming increase in cancers, premature death and in mental and physical deficiencies among adults and children! Three generations now show the effects of being reared on this "junk food" diet and its dramatic increase in hyperactive and violent youngsters.

169

Official estimates reveal that about 5% of American children are afflicted with minimal brain dysfunction as the result of pollutants in our food, water and air! This tragic fact, combined with the steady increase of mental and emotional disturbances among adults of all ages, is reminding the medical profession of the basic precept of its founder, Hippocrates: **Let food be your medicine.**

Nervous Problems are Epidemic!

In our hectic world there is often so much pressure to stay on the go that we forget how to relax. We've met many people over the years who never took time to slow down and smell the roses! These people never take breaks from their stressful lives until it's too late – working, rushing and worrying until their health deteriorates.

Happiness is not being pained in body or troubled in mind.
– Thomas Jefferson, 3rd U.S. President, 1797-1801

It's magnificent to live long if one keeps healthy, youthful and active.
– Harry Emerson Fosdick, American Clergyman (1878-1969)

Old age is not a time of life. It is a condition of the body. It is not time that ages the body, it is abuse that does! – Herbert M. Shelton

It's no wonder that modern medicine is reporting epidemics in nervous disorders. Medical conditions like Attention Deficit Hyperactivity Disorders (ADHD) and Chronic Fatigue Syndrome (CFS), which were almost unheard of until recently, are now common diagnoses. In fact, according to National Institute of Mental Health, there are now over 17 million Americans suffering from ADHD alone and 4 million ADHD victims are children! Sad Facts!!!

Many Youngsters Have Stress Too

A *New York Times/CBS News* poll found teenagers aged 13 to 17, from affluent homes regardless of race or gender, had more stress than those from modest homes. Wealthy youngsters often have less perspective on struggles of life, but there's pressure to keep family's status – getting into elite schools, good grades and living up to parents' academic expectations, etc. A Christian home life can help guide teenagers with life's stresses.

Attention Deficit Hyperactivity Disorder

ADHD is not caused by bugs or disease. There is no laboratory test that can identify it. ADHD is a condition brought on by depleted and exhausted nerves. People with ADHD live at a low rate of vibration – the victims of a weakened Nerve Force. They have little energy to pay attention, to complete tasks or to ward off worry and frustration. Doctors, teachers and psychiatrists prescribe drugs like Ritalin at an ever increasing rate.

Although over 8 million school children are taking Ritalin, ADHD is still the fastest growing childhood disorder in U.S.! Drugs might mask some symptoms of Nerve Depletion, but do not replenish Nerve Force. Not surprisingly, more studies are finding that drugs are a dead-end in the treatment of ADHD! Instead, they are finding that people are renewed to health only when they follow a healthy lifestyle that replenishes their reserves of Nerve Force. ADHD sufferers need to

---

Ritalin is sadly most commonly prescribed psychostimulant. It works by increasing the activity of the central nervous system. The benefits and cost effectiveness of Ritalin long term are unknown due to lack of research! The long term effects on the developing brain are unknown. Ritalin is not approved for children under six years of age. See www.mercola.com.

build up their Nerve Force. This is accomplished, not through drugs, but through the kinds of changes in diet and lifestyle that we outline in this book. Australian researchers found ADHD children began replenishing their Nerve Force after they were put on a natural diet free of coloring, preservatives, sugars, etc. A similar study by the Cornell Medical Center recorded a 73% improvement with ADHD patients.

Unnatural and altered foods tax the nervous system, as do highly sweetened and processed foods! Children are at a greater risk of harm from this kind of diet! As our foods become more processed and refined, our children become inattentive, unfocused, unhealthy and unhappy!

Nutritional Therapy Brings Miracles For Hyperactive and Challenged Children

Even more than the non-responsive "challenged" child, the hyperkinetic slow learner or "hyperactive under-achiever" is becoming a more common serious problem today. These children are characterized by almost continuous irrational behavior, very short attention span and difficulty in comprehension. A number of research studies report that children in both categories are now responding with great improvement with nutritional supplement therapy. Most notable are efforts of the New York Institute for Child Development (with a record of more than 1,500 cases) and – in San Francisco – at the Kaiser-Permanente Hospital's Allergy Clinic, the famous study directed by Dr. Benjamin Feingold (see web: *www.feingold.org*). An individualized program of diet and exercise is prescribed after a series of biochemical and neurological tests.

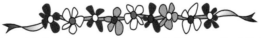

When Dr. Feingold first began to use diet (then called K-P diet) to treat children with ADHD (then called hyperkinesis), he said that 30% to 50% of the children got better. Later, after he eliminated the petrochemical preservatives BHA and BHT (TBHQ didn't exist yet), he found that over 70% of the children got better. We still see that same – or better – result today. About 50% of children (or adults) don't need any other intervention. The others still need more help, which may be educational adjustments, tutoring, supplements, further restrictions due to identified allergies, behavior modification or counseling. – See web: feingold.org/adhd.php

Here is Dr. Feingold's Basic Health Program:

1. Elimination of all refined sugar, refined flour products and all foods containing toxic additives, caffeine, preservatives and artificial sweeteners and coloring.

2. High protein (preferably vegetarian), low carbohydrate meals with an emphasis on fresh, raw organic fruits, vegetables and their fresh juices.

3. Natural vitamin and mineral food supplements – especially B6 and the other B vitamins, vitamin C, E, niacin, pantothenic acid, magnesium and calcium – plus others determined for patient's needs.

In other words, this is basically the same nutritional program we have been advocating for 4 generations! The same diet – combined with generous doses of vitamins and minerals – is being used successfully in the treatment of children with serious brain damage at the Institute for the Achievement of Human Potential in Philadelphia, PA.

In Dr. Feingold's book, *An Introduction to Clinical Allergy,* showed two companion graphs covering the ten year study that demonstrated the parallel between the yearly sales of artificial sweeteners (such as aspartame, NutraSweet, etc., see page 177), and soft drinks and the increase of hyperkinesia (hyperactivity), anger and learning difficulties among children in the United States.

Chronic Fatigue Syndrome – CFS

CFS, like ADHD, is not a disease. It is a condition in which fatigue and tiredness rule the heart and minds of its victims. These people live at a low rate of vibration which makes their normal life seem a burden. When life's small tasks become great exertions, what then are life's challenges? Clearly, chronic fatigue is a quality of life destroyer that must be understood and overcome.

Back in the 1980's, CFS was called the "Yuppie Flu," a relatively rare condition that affected mostly the upper middle class. Now researchers at DePaul University (*cfids.org*), have shattered that image. They found that as many as 800,000 people nationwide may suffer from CFS, twice the number previously estimated by Atlanta's Center for Disease Control and Prevention. The study estimated that Chronic Fatigue Syndrome was found in 183 cases per 100,000 persons ages 18-69. The highest rates of CFS were found among Caucasian women – 522 per 100,000. In men, 291 per 100,000 had CFS. This study indicated that CFS affects women and men of all racial and ethnic groups, as well as adolescents. However, Caucasian women have the highest risk for CFS. The risk of getting CFS is considerably higher than that of getting lung cancer – 63 per 100,000. (*www.cfids.org*).

These are the symptoms for CFS: debilitating fatigue, impairment of short-term memory or concentration, sore throat, tender lymph nodes, muscle and joint pain, headaches, unrefreshing sleep and fatigue lasting more than 24 hours following exertion. To be diagnosed with CFS, a person must have had these symptoms for more than six months and not be diagnosed with any other medical illness or ailments. Many CFS patients are unable to hold jobs, attend school or care for their family.

CFS Healing Testimony for Bragg Healthy Lifestyle

Diagnosed with Chronic Fatigue Syndrome, Fibromyalgia, Clinical and Manic Depression, I have been on every drug imaginable and tried every Doctor-type treatment recommended – but only got worse! In the last 6-8 months I changed my diet, began exercising and discontinued ALL medications. I have been living the Bragg Healthy Lifestyle including a weekly 24 hour fast. I feel incredible – sinus headaches and bloating gone. I am more focused and directed. Depression, fatigue, body tension – all gone! I have my life back – I am in control of my health and life! I got back to basics with the Bragg Health Books and Healthy Lifestyle. Patricia, you truly are a Crusading Angel and make such a difference in so many people's lives. God Bless you – thank you! – Marilyn, CA

Some therapies tried by people with chronic fatigue syndrome include: massage therapy, acupuncture, chiropractic therapy, self-hypnosis, and therapeutic touch. People with CFS may feel better with such techniques, but these therapies should be combined with an individualized exercise program that includes stretching. – see web: www.emedicinehealth.com

The doctor of the future will no longer treat the human frame with drugs, but rather will cure and prevent disease with nutrition. – Thomas Edison

May food be your medicine. The natural healing force within us is the greatest force in getting well. – Hippocrates, Father of Medicine, 400 B.C.

There is truth in the saying that man becomes what he eats. – Gandhi

A strong, healthy body makes the mind strong.
– Thomas Jefferson, 3rd U.S. President, 1797-1801

Dr. James Balch's Health Suggestions to Combat Chronic Fatigue Syndrome*:

- Eat a well-balanced, natural, healthy diet of 50% raw, organically grown foods and fresh "live" juices. The diet should consist mostly of fruits, vegetables, whole grains, plus raw nuts, seeds, skinless turkey and some deep-water fish. These quality foods supply nutrients that renew energy and help build your immunity.

- Add some form of acidophilus to your diet, and regularly consume soured products like soy yogurt, sauerkraut, yogurt, kefir, etc. Many people with chronic fatigue syndrome also are infected with candida. Acidophilus helps to keep candida under control.

- Drink distilled water – at least 8 glasses per day, plus freshly made fruit and vegetable juices. Water flushes out toxins and helps reduce muscle and joint pain.

- Do not eat shellfish, fried foods, junk foods, processed refined foods, sugar and white flour products – desserts, bread and pasta, and stay away from stimulants – coffee, black tea and cola drinks – see *foods to avoid list* on page 101.

- Add ample fiber to your diet and make sure that the bowels move daily. Give yourself occasional enemas.

- Take chlorophyll in liquid or tablet form and take protein supplements or powders from a vegetable source such as Spirulina or Barley Green.

- Certain amino acids may be beneficial for those with CFS, they include: tyrosine, leucine, isoleucine, valine, lysine and taurine.

- Get plenty of rest. Make sure you don't over-exert yourself. Melatonin is helpful for promoting restful sleep. Skullcap and valerian root also improve sleep.

Amino acids are needed for building every part of the body: bones, blood, hair, skin, nails and glands, etc. – are Mother Nature's and God's life-giving secret for a long, vital life. – Paul C. Bragg, N.D., Ph.D.

---

*Dr. James Balch, in "Prescription for Nutritional Healing" states: CFS can cause serious damage to your immune system. You must combat it.

- Try a variety of teas from burdock root, dandelion, red clover and Pau d'Arco. The Bragg Organic Apple Cider Vinegar Drink also helps promote healing.

- Ginkgo Biloba, St. John's Wort and SAMe are also beneficial for those with Chronic Fatigue Syndrome.

- Taking echinacea and goldenseal enhances immune function and helps with cold and flu symptoms.

- Other important nutrients are: CoQ10, calcium, lecithin, potassium, malic acid, magnesium, manganese, vitamins A, B, C, E, zinc, garlic, black currant, primrose oil capsules, and maitake or shiitake reishi mushrooms available fresh or dried (soak ½ hour before eating) or in caps and powders.

For more on chronic fatigue and CFIDS see web: *cfids.org*

Avoiding Metabolic Syndrome

Metabolic Syndrome is regarded as a collection of disease risk factors caused by insulin resistance, which pre-disposes you to diabetes, heart disease and stroke. **175** A recent study (*mercola.com*) has found a correlation between the lack of micronutrients such as folate, zinc and vitamins B12, C, E and D. To boost your metabolism, it is important to eliminate sugar and excess salt in your meals; exercise regularly and get adequate amounts of sleep.

Your biological rhythm of sleeping and awaking is known as circadian rhythm – this is intricately tied to your metabolism. If you deprive yourself of adequate sleep, you disrupt your metabolism. Lack of sleep also affects your levels of leptin and ghrelin – two hormones linked with appetite and eating. When you are sleep deprived, your body decreases production of leptin, the hormone that tells your brain that you are not hungry. At the same time, it increases your levels of ghrelin – a hormone that triggers hunger! This results in a weak and sluggish metabolism. The right amount of sleep is based on your own individual needs. See pages 67-80.

Exercising, along with weight training, eating a healthy diet, getting some healthy, gentle sunshine, along with solid sleeping habits can go a long way toward optimizing your metabolism.

For fast-acting relief, try slowing down. – Lily Tomlin, comedian

Diet is Vital to Developing Intelligence and Brain Cells

To prove that proper nutrition is effective not only for restoring normality to children with brain dysfunctions, but also for increasing learning ability of children considered normal, New York Institute for Child Development tested the effect of controlled foods and vitamins on children in Harlem nurseries. There was a 20% increase in their I.Q.'s over 1 year! Similar studies in other parts of the country have also confirmed these findings. For example, a psychological study by M. B. Stoch and P. M. Smythe, compared undernourished children with properly nourished children from similar backgrounds and parentage, discovered a 22 I.Q. points difference in favor of the well nourished children over a period of years!

"All the learning opportunities in the world will be of no avail, unless infants are at the same time furnished with everything they need to build up their brain cell structures," states Dr. Roger J. Williams in *Nutrition Against Disease* (*amazon.com*). He also stresses that the brain is strongly vulnerable to malnutrition and its effects. **In 1998 Salk Institute in La Jolla, CA, found in their landmark study that humans can generate new brain cells (see: *www.salk.edu*).**

"Junk Foods" Starve the Brain and Body

These studies all focus on the harmful food additives, white flour and excessive sugar, as the primary culprits that upset the normal functioning of the brain. These, of course, are the basic ingredients of the "junk food" diet that most young Americans are raised on; empty calorie foodless foods. All the essential nourishment, including vitamins, minerals and other nutrients, have been "refined" out. No so-called "enrichment" with synthetic vitamins can replace natural, healthy nutrition. Dr. Feingold pointed out, some of the most harmful toxic additives are now being used in synthetic vitamins, and especially in those brands widely advertised for children!

The biochemical tests on hyperactive children show they suffer from vitamin, mineral, and enzyme deficiencies and imbalances and also from hypoglycemia. It's ironic that hypoglycemia or low blood sugar, is most often the result of the over-consumption of refined white sugar and its products (such as candy, ice cream, cola drinks, etc.) and refined white flour products (pizzas, pastries, donuts, etc.) which are converted into empty calories in the body.

This excessive amount of sugar over-stimulates the production of insulin by the pancreas as a result of the natural biochemical reaction to rid the body of the excess sugar, but the empty sugar calories are so quickly consumed that the extra insulin then depletes the body's natural sugar as well. This causes the blood sugar to drop below normal, which creates an appetite for even more sugar! Unless the hypoglycemic's diet is effectively controlled, this vicious circle keeps on repeating itself.

The brain suffers from low blood sugar more than any other part of the body. Although other organs can derive energy from various sources, the brain depends almost exclusively on the oxidation of glucose (the energy substance of sugar). Hypoglycemia starves the brain, and when you starve the brain, you starve the control "computer" center of the individual human being!

Stevia – Natural Herbal Sweetener

Stevia is an herb native to South America. It is widely grown for its sweet leaves. In its unprocessed form it is 30 times sweeter than sugar. It is a low carbohydrate, low-sugar food alternative. Stevia shows promise for treating such conditions as obesity and high blood pressure. It does not effect blood sugar and it even enhances glucose tolerance. Stevia makes a safe, delicious, health sweetener for diabetics. Children can use Stevia without concerns as it does not cause cavities.

Beware of Deadly Aspartame Sugar Substitutes!

Although its name sounds "tame," this deadly neurotoxin is anything but! Aspartame is an artificial sweetener (over 200 times sweeter than sugar) made by Monsanto Corporation and marketed as "NutraSweet," "Equal," "Spoonful," and countless other trade names. Although aspartame is added to over 9,000 food products, it is not fit for human consumption! This toxic poison changes into formaldehyde in the body and has been linked to migraines, seizures, vision loss and symptoms relating to lupus, Parkinson's Disease, Multiple Sclerosis and other health destroying conditions (even Gulf War Syndrome). For more info on this toxic killer – this crime against our health, check webs: aspartamekills.com *and* holisticmed.com/aspartame.

Hypoglycemia and Violence On Rise

Violent behavior in all ages often is a symptom of hypoglycemia (page 8). Violent behavior of hyperactive youth has been biochemically identified as deriving from hypoglycemia. This antisocial behavior has been reversed and returned to normal by proper diet (page 171-172).

What about the increasingly tragic high incidence of "unprovoked violence" among teens and young adults? With increasing drug and alcohol addiction and other symptoms of diet deficiencies, violence ranging from vandalism to murder is epidemic and occurring in affluent as well as poverty-ridden areas. The common denominator among these young people is their "junk food" high sugar diet! So far, medical research has not explored this field, but an ethnographer (a specialist in descriptive anthropology) has recently reported findings which reveal a connection.

178 Ralph Bolton, an ethnographer from Pomona College in Claremont, California, and his wife, Charlene, were prompted by medical reports of violent behavior as a common symptom of hypoglycemia to investigate this phenomenon as it pertained to human society. As the subject of their study they selected the Qolla, an isolated tribe in the Andes Mountains of Peru. For four centuries – ever since they were first discovered by Spanish explorers – this tribe has been recognized as among the most dangerously aggressive people in the world.

The Boltons bravely spent two years among Qolla tribes, whom they found to be simple and essentially good people, but quick to anger, irrationally violent and given to murderous rages. They also found the Qolla diet to be excessively high in sugar! Consumption begins in the early morning when the village candy salesman makes his rounds, and continues throughout the day along with the drinking of alcohol and chewing of coca leaves (which stimulates glucose levels).

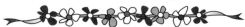

*Everyone thinks of changing the world,
but seldom thinks of changing himself.*

Violence and anger inhibits peace, health and spiritual growth.

With the cooperation of local physicians, controlled tests were made for hypoglycemia. Also a secret ballot poll was taken in the village as to who among the villagers were rated as the most violent. More than half of those tested had hypoglycemia and these individuals were the same ones who were voted by their peers as being the most violent! A check of legal records bore this out, since all the hypoglycemics had been involved in violent antisocial behavior and accused of homicide! In his report, Bolton speculates that violent behavior might well be a natural biochemical reaction in hypoglycemia. He believes that the body's attempts to restore the blood sugar balance by stimulating the production of adrenaline – which in turn triggers the liver to produce glucose – lead to the Qolla's antisocial angered behavior. The theory is logical.

It seems logical to us to start testing this theory of dietary influence on the aggressive behavior in all the "corrective" Institutions in America which "incorrigible" juveniles and young adults are confined. From all reports, the meals are predominantly starch, with an abundance of refined flour products and "treats" made with refined white sugar. A change to the diet that has been so effective with hyperkinetic children could work wonders! These young people could participate in healthy exercise by raising their own healthy organically grown fruits and vegetables. The physical and psychological effects could accomplish genuine miracle reform, the alleged purpose of Institutions to make them good citizens!

Vitamin and Mineral Food Supplements in the Treatment of Mental Illness

The biochemical-nutritional approach is making headway in that last frontier of medicine: mental illness. Many leading psychiatrists today are convinced that a physical cause can be found for various mental disorders and diseases. Since 1959, the Brain Research Institute at University of California at Los Angeles (UCLA) has worked intensively to analyze the biochemistry of depression and other mental illnesses to discover the effect of dietary deficiencies on mental health and how these can be corrected. Amazing results are happening (ucla.edu).

At the N.J. Psychiatric Institute, famous Dr. Carl C. Pfeiffer has found that one form of schizophrenia (known as "mauve-positive") responds to treatment with specific vitamin and mineral food supplements. He reported on the case of a 15-year-old schizophrenic patient who has been returned to, and maintained normalcy for 2 years, on daily supplements of 1,000 mgs of vitamin B6, and some zinc and manganese. When these supplements were discontinued in a test, the patient relapsed into her schizophrenic state (convulsions, insomnia, etc.). Now, in situations which may cause stress, she simply increases her daily quota of B6 (500 to 800 mgs)! There are other reports of similar cases that responded to massive supplements of B6, and niacin (B3).

Medicine treats symptoms, while nutrition treats causes,

– declared by Dr. Grace Song Line – a nutritional therapy pioneer – who dramatically demonstrated this principal early in her career. A native of Korea, she came to the United States after obtaining her medical degree in Japan. In 1929 she became the first woman in the U.S. to receive a degree as Doctor of Public Health. At the Michigan State Mental Hospital, Dr. Line took over the treatment of a "hopeless" case – a 20 year old girl who was unable to eat or take care of herself in any way and was being milk-fed by tube. Dr. Line stopped the milk-feeding and the electric shock treatments to which the girl had been subjected. She then put the patient on condensed liver broth supplemented by massive doses of niacinamide, plus other natural multi-vitamins and minerals fed to her through the tube, as well as a daily intravenous injection of vital B-Complex, niacinamide B3 and B12. Amazingly, within a week the girl was taking care of herself (dressing, combing her hair, etc.), developed a normal appetite and could feed herself. The doctors at the hospital pronounced it "miraculous".

Dr. Line continued such "miracles" using nutritional therapy throughout a lifetime of treating degenerative diseases in patients of all ages. Along with therapeutic doses of supplemental vitamins and minerals, she insisted on a diet of strictly organic, chemical-free foods and pure water!

Magnesium – Essential for Healthy Nerves

The vital role of magnesium in the treatment of certain emotional and mental disorders – ranging from mental fatigue to frightening hallucinations – was not detected until very recently because magnesium levels are usually measured by sampling the blood serum. Two physicians – Dr. Richard C. W. Hall of the U.S. Naval Hospital in Orlando, Florida and Dr. Joy R. Joffe of Johns Hopkins University College of Medicine – have discovered that blood serum levels can remain normal while magnesium levels in the brain and cerebrospinal fluid may be dangerously low. This discovery has clarified previous confusion in attempts to correlate magnesium deficiency with a variety of symptoms that indicate degeneration of nerve, brain and heart tissue. Today these complications – which often appear in connection with certain conditions such as alcoholism, severe burns, chronic diarrhea, malnutrition in infants and adults, arrhythmia, etc. – are being treated successfully with magnesium orotate or sulfate, given orally or by injection.

181

Although serious magnesium deficiencies can be fatal, even a minor deficiency of this vital mineral can cause personality changes. What some doctors call the *housewife syndrome*; i.e. a general lassitude, low back pain, tension headaches, an excessive desire to sleep, but inability to sleep soundly, lack of interest in home duties and the marital relationship, has been remedied within a week's time with magnesium, calcium and potassium supplements (available Health Stores).

To assure the healthy functioning of your nerves and brain, be sure to include good sources of organic magnesium, such as nuts of all kinds (raw is best), non-hydrogenated peanut and nut butters, organic steel-cut oatmeal, raw sesame seeds, soybeans, stone-ground cornmeal, whole wheat flour, organic spinach, avocado, beans and especially raw wheat germ in your diet.

Natural vitamins, minerals and food supplements are good insurance factors in helping to keep the body well nourished, peaceful and healthy.

Magnesium is a superstar nutrient that plays a role in approximately 300 vital functions in the body. – Life Extension Magazine (www.lef.org)

75 % of Adults Deficient in Magnesium

A recent report by the World Health Organization found that 75% of adult Americans were eating less than the RDA (Recommended Dietary Allowance) of magnesium. They also found that magnesium consumption tends to decrease with age. *"Magnesium deficiency is a concern for all ages, but for the elderly, it could be particularly serious,"* says Richard Rivlin, M.D., Chief Nutrition Division of New York Hospital – Cornell Medical Center (*medicalnewstoday.com*)

Magnesium is one of the body's major electrolytes, along with potassium, calcium and sodium. It is involved in over 300 enzymatic reactions in the body, and is vital for the proper functioning of the heart and nervous system. Causes for magnesium depletion include: use of birth control pills, excessive use of alcohol, a diet of refined foods and stress. Researchers believe that stress causes magnesium to be released from the cells and then excreted in the urine. Many health practitioners have found that supplementing with magnesium, rather than prescribing tranquilizers, is what is needed for those who suffer from this nervousness, restless leg syndrome, ADHD, irritability, anxiety, or depression. Studies also showed that, along with magnesium (orotate or sulfate is best), that also vitamin B6 helps ease symptoms of premenstrual syndrome.

How Much Magnesium Do You Need?

RDA for magnesium is 350 mgs for men and 300 mgs for women. Pregnant or nursing women require an extra 150 mgs. Though magnesium naturally occurs in most raw foods, a healthy daily amount of 350 mgs is hard to attain eating processed and junk foods. Eat organic apples, apricots, avocados, bananas, green leafy vegetables, garlic, beans, soybeans, soy products, raw nuts and seeds, brown rice, tofu, whole wheat and other whole grains, which are rich in magnesium. Herbs such as cayenne, alfalfa, fennel, hops and paprika also add magnesium.

Take 1,000 mgs of calcium daily in conjunction with 500 mgs of magnesium daily. Postmenopausal women are advised to take 1,500 mgs calcium. Choose a calcium formula that contains mixed compounds such as citrate, carbonate, aspartate and gluconate in combination with similar magnesium complex. – see: drsinatra.com

Only 25% of Americans consume the Recommended Daily Allowance (RDA) amount. Mildred Seelig, M.D., has spent years researching magnesium and is the world authority on the subject. Dr. Seelig recommends an intake of at least 6 mg per kilogram of body weight. This would mean 300 mg for a 100-pound person, 420 mg for a 154-pound person, and 540 mg for a 200-pound person. Shari Lieberman, M.S., R.D. suggests that the optimal daily allowance for both men and women should be 500 – 750 mg daily. People with osteoporosis, high blood pressure, arrhythmia or angina, or women taking oral contraceptives, should take even higher levels, says Lieberman. Magnesium supplementing should be properly balanced to include correct levels of calcium, zinc and potassium. Robert K. Rude, M.D., of the Southern California School of Medicine, finds that magnesium deficiency is associated with low blood levels of calcium and potassium. Dr. Rude says that magnesium should be used in lower amounts cautiously by those that have impaired kidney function.

Calcium: The Other Half of the Dynamic Duo

Calcium is important too, because of its synergistic relationship with magnesium. Although most people associate calcium deficits with poor bone health, low levels can also increase your vulnerability to high blood pressure. But you must be careful about the amount of calcium you take. More than 2,000 mg of calcium per day can cause your kidneys to excrete magnesium!

Chelation Therapy Cleanses Arteries

As discussed earlier, organic calcium is essential for maintaining the health of the brain, heart and nervous system. However, inorganic calcium can be deadly! It can't be absorbed or assimilated by the body and is therefore deposited in joints (arthritis), especially along the artery walls. There it not only hardens arteries and makes them brittle, but also collects deposits of excess cholesterol, forming plaques that clog and impede flow of blood. Chelation Therapy helps remove these plaques.

Cheerfulness is the atmosphere under which all things thrive. – Jean Paul Richter

Within the last thirty years this process known as Chelation Therapy has been carefully developed which removes these abnormal deposits of inorganic calcium from arterial walls and other parts of the body without disturbing the normal balance of organic calcium. Results have been termed "miraculous" by physicians as well as patients. We discuss Chelation Therapy in detail in our book *Healthy Heart and Cardiovascular System*. See back pages for ordering this Bragg book.

The number of Chelation Clinics around the world is growing. In America, for a list of Chelation Doctors contact:

American College of Advancement in Medicine, 24411 Ridge Route, #115, Laguna Hills, CA 92653 Referral Hotline: Call (888) 439-6891 See website: *www.acam.org*

In Europe, we met with world famous Dr. Claus Martin who has the vision, wisdom and education to direct his lovely *Four Seasons Clinic* in the Bavarian Alps that provides chelation, oxygen, and live cell therapy from March to November. These are remarkable life-prolonging treatments that can help reverse the age-related and degenerative cardiovascular diseases. Hollywood Stars, Famous Statesmen and other noteworthy people have and are reaping the benefits of his treatments. He is a long time highly respected member of ACAM. There are over 200 chelation clinics throughout Europe. Checkout ACAM website or if in Europe write or call:

Dr. Claus Martin, M.D., Four Seasons Clinic Box 244, D-83700 Rottach-Egern, Germany PHONE: 011-49-8022-26780; FAX 011-49-8022-24740

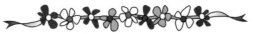

We must always change, renew, rejuvenate; otherwise, we harden. – Goethe

---

It's good that modern technology is available if you need it, but it's even better to prevent your arteries from getting plugged up in the first place.

Health Stores now have oral chelation supplements and Niacin (B3), etc.

Physically fit people live longer and enjoy a better quality of life. – Tedd Mitchell, M.D., Cooper Clinic, www.cooperaerobics.com

---

A light, happy heart lives longer. – William Shakespeare

Healthy Body = More Peaceful Mind

- Everybody feels happier when they are looking good and taking a multi vitamin and mineral food supplements. They contribute specifically to your health and good looks!

- Vitamin D contributes to the strength and density of bones. A lack of vitamin D can lead to osteoporosis, which often affects the posture, reason oldsters do better with some "vitamin D's sunshine" and a good multi-mineral with calcium, boron and magnesium. Also get 15 minutes of gentle sun exposure a few times a week, preferably early or late sun (see pages 147-148).

- Vitamin A contributes to healthy skin, hair, eyes and strong, durable bones and tooth enamel.

- The B vitamins – niacin, riboflavin, B6, B12 and also magnesium help to prevent growth retardation in young people. Niacin and riboflavin help prevent skin rashes, lip sores and lip cracks and protects your nerves.

185

- Vitamin B complex promotes normal functioning of the brain and helps in resistance to stress.

- Folic acid plays a vital role in the smooth functioning of a healthy body, it improves brain function, helps lessen depression, anxiety and lowers homocysteine levels. In addition to supplements, folic acid is found in dates, Bragg Nutritional Yeast and broccoli (page 88).

- Vitamin C (and Ester C) is a powerful antioxidant which fights diseases, colds, flu, etc. (including cancer) and helps prevent high blood pressure and blood clotting. It's vital for tissue growth and repair (especially bruising), helps reduce cholesterol levels and increases the absorption of the mineral iron.

All vitamins and minerals listed above, and many more which are found naturally in the Bragg Healthy Lifestyle Diet will help you maintain a healthier, happier body and a more peaceful mind!

Anxiety, stress and insomnia are some of the most troublesome problems people treat with conventional medicine. The drugs used have many side effects, and most are habit forming. Natural remedies provide a safe, healthier alternative and are becoming the first treatment of choice.
– Rob McCaleb, Herb Research Foundation

Mother Nature Loves You To Enjoy Her Beauty

186

Let me look upward
into the branches
Of the towering oak
And know that it grew
slowly and well.

Give me, amidst
the confusion
of my day
The calmness of the
everlasting hills.

Let me pause
to look at a flower,
to smell a rose —
God's autograph,
to chat with a friend,
to read a few lines
from a good book.

Break the tensions
of my nerves
With the soothing music
of singing streams
and gentle rains
That live in
my memory.

Follow steps of the Godly,
and stay on the right path
to enjoy life to the fullest.
– Proverbs 2:20-21

Mother Nature and friendships are cozy shelters for life's rainy days.

Chapter 14

Relief is on the Way for Nervous Tension, Stress and Anxiety

Here's One of the Main Causes of Nervous Tension, Stress and Anxiety

Amazingly nervous tension, stress and anxiety are caused often by an increased production of hormone-producing glands, including the thyroid, parathyroid, adrenals, thymus, hypothalamus, pituitary as well as the ovaries and testes. The hormones of the endocrine glands work to keep the body in a state of normal balance, acting chemically on the body organs to keep growth, appetite, blood pressure, heart rate, sexual drive, and other bodily processes running smoothly. *"Certain glands have more functions than others,"* explains Dr. Mark Gold, author of *The Good News About Panic, Anxiety & Phobias (amazon.com). "The tiny hypothalamus acts as a master gland, regulating all the body's processes, from the sleep/wake cycle to heart rate, hunger and emotions. When it seems unbalanced, it orders the appropriate gland to produce the needed level of the correct hormone to reestablish equilibrium."* Most endocrine problems arise when a particular gland fails to produce the proper amount of hormone. The brain notices the imbalance immediately, and the mind, emotions and behavior can all be affected.

Almost all body functions and organs react to nervous tension, stress and anxiety. The pituitary gland increases its production of adrenal hormones, which in turn stimulates the release of the hormones, cortisone and cortisol. These have the effect of inhibiting the functioning of disease-fighting white blood cells and suppressing the immune response. Increased adrenaline production causes the body to step up its metabolism of protein, fats, and carbohydrates to quickly produce energy for the body to use. This response causes the body to store less calcium, excrete vital amino acids, potassium

187

and phosphorus and depletes magnesium stored in muscle tissue. The body does not absorb ingested nutrients well when under stress, nervous tension or anxiety and therefore becomes deficient in many nutrients. Nervous tension, stress and anxiety also promote the formation of free radicals that can become oxidized and damage body tissues, especially cell membranes. Researchers have found that nearly 80% of all major illnesses, including cardiovascular disease, cancer, endocrine and metabolic diseases, skin disorders, back problems and other physical ailments, are believed to be related to stress, nervous tension and anxiety. B-complex vitamins are very helpful for proper functioning of the nervous system. Anti-stress enzymes such as L-Tyrosine, as well as calcium, zinc, magnesium, melatonin, SAMe, ginkgo biloba, and St. John's Wort are also helpful (see pages 193-194, 197).

Chronic Depression May Lead to Cancer

According to researchers at the National Institute on Ageing in Bethesda, they tracked 4,825 elderly Americans for 10 years, and found that those who were chronically depressed during the first six years of the study were almost twice as likely to develop cancer as their non-depressed counter-parts. (See web: *depression.net*) Cancer malignancies of the breast, colon, lung and prostate were prominent in chronically depressed individuals. The researchers stated that depression cannot be considered a cause for cancer, but they noted that depression boosts blood levels of stress hormones, which impair immune function. Chronic depression appears to suppress the immune system significantly enough and long enough to allow cancer cells to multiply. You may seek on-line psychotherapy by contacting: *www.psychotherapy.net* or seek medical information by contacting *medsurf.com*.

Link Between Stress and Cancer

According to Scientists at the National Cancer Institute (*cancer.gov*); psychological stress can affect the immune system, your body's defense against diseases such as cancer. Your body responds to stress by releasing hormones such as adrenalin and cortisol which help you react to a stressful situation by giving you more strength and speed. However, stress hormones increase your blood pressure, heart rate, and blood sugar levels.

Prolonged chronic stress can dangerously increase your risk for obesity; depression; and abuse of drugs and alcohol. Studies also found that chronic stress can affect cancer tumor growth and weaken your immune system.

Importance of Normalizing Blood Pressure

A recent Mayo Clinic study found nearly 40% of the participants who had high blood pressure were unaware of their condition, and only 17% of those with the problem had it under control. Researchers were especially concerned because these participants lived in prosperous communities and had easy access to health care. When left untreated, *this silent killer* – high blood pressure increases a person's risk for heart disease, stroke and kidney failure. Although high blood pressure is predominant in men; after the age of 55 – men and women are at equal risk! Blood pressure is the force of blood against the vessel walls. Systolic pressure is the pressure of the blood in the vessels as the heart beats. Diastolic pressure is the pressure of the blood between heartbeats. If your systolic pressure is 140 or above, and diastolic pressure is 90 or above, it is considered high. Unfortunately, high blood pressure has no symptoms, so it's important to have your blood pressure checked regularly.

189

To aid in lowering your blood pressure follow these important tips: Lose excess weight; increase physical activity that helps strengthen heart, blood vessels and helps you lose weight. Exercise 30 minutes daily; reduce sodium (salt) in your diet; limit or better yet, stop alcohol – it harms the body, brain, etc. and raises blood pressure, plus adds unnecessary calories. Increase your potassium intake – found in fruits, vegetables and Bragg's Organic Apple Cider Vinegar. Potassium helps to normalize blood pressure and the body's vital acid/alkaline balance.

CoQ10 Combats Heart Disease, Cancer, Gum Disease and Ageing:

- *90-120 mgs daily as preventive in cardiovascular or periodontal disease*
- *120 to 240 mgs CoQ10 daily for angina pectoris, high blood pressure, cardiac arrhythmia and gingivitis (gum disease)*
- *240-450 mgs daily for congestive heart failure & dilated cardiomyopathy*
  – Dr. Stephen T. Sinatra, author, *CoQ10 Phenomenon* • sinatramd.com

High blood pressure can lead to decline in some mental abilities, according to researchers at the University of Maine. Elevated blood pressure is a strong predictor of changes in brain structure and related cognitive functioning.

Hypertension Can Be Prevented

According to Scientists, they found we all carry a salt gene, called angiotensinogen, that can affect our blood pressure. Those with mutated forms of this gene are more likely to develop high blood pressure, say Researchers in the *Hypertension Journal* (*www.elsevier.com*). Blood pressure declines in people with this altered gene when they use less salt. American Heart Assoc. recommends no more than 2,400 mgs of sodium daily. Bragg Liquid Aminos is a delicious all-purpose seasoning that contains less than 110 mg organic sodium per ½ tsp and is a safe salt substitute.

Read labels! All cured meats (salami, bacon, hot dogs, etc.), frozen dinners, canned foods, soups, chilis, etc. and pretzels, chips, and snack foods contain lots of salt. Sweets such as cookies, cakes and soft drinks are loaded with sodium and sugar – best to avoid them! Instead, consume lots of calcium and potassium rich foods; both of these minerals have healthy beneficial effects on blood pressure. Bragg's Apple Cider Vinegar is a healthy source of potassium! For further hypertension information check these websites: *Medicinenet.com, www.nhlbi.nih.gov/hbp/index.html* and *www.lifeclinic.com*

Combating Depression, Stress & Anxiety

According to the American Psychiatric Association, the good news about depression is that it's more treatable than ever. It's common to get *the blues* when you are disappointed or lose a job or a loved one. However, when diagnosed accurately, there's virtually no one who can't be helped, says Dr. John McIntyre, of APA. Patients who have used long-term antidepressant prescription drugs found these drugs cause side-effects of drowsiness, insomnia, headaches, nausea and other gastrointestinal symptoms. There are many non-drug therapies available now to combat depression that have no side-effects.

"Herbal medicines can be effective in treating anxiety and stress, but they work best when they are part of a natural self-healing program", notes Dr. Harold H. Bloomfield, author of *Healing Anxiety with Herbs* (*amazon.com*). Kava Herbal Extract is a natural tranquilizer, and as effective as the drug Benzodiazepine Serax (Oxazepam).

Kava is a member of the pepper tree family and is used widely in Europe for treating anxiety and insomnia. Other helpful herbs are: St. John's Wort, SAMe, Valerian, Chamomile, California Poppy, Hops, Passion Flower, Ginseng, Milk Thistle, Ginkgo Biloba, Licorice Root, Ashwagandha, Reishi Mushrooms and Rauwolfia Serpentina. Do seek sound health advice and the treatment which will bring you the best health results!

Researchers have shown that those who enjoy a healthy active lifestyle are the most resistant to stress and anxiety! An active lifestyle that includes 30 minutes or more of daily exercise; stretching your muscles and body to allow a natural open flow of energy; eating healthy nutritional meals; and if possible do put in a herb and veggie garden, it's good fun!

More Stress Relieving Suggestions:

- Gardening – researchers have found that to garden helps relieve tensions and is a powerful natural medicine for emotional, spiritual and physical healing.

- Enjoying natural beauty – scientific studies indicate that when individuals view beautiful natural scenes such as waterfalls, trees, animals, flowers, etc., they relieve anxiety, relax more easily and feel happier.

- Reduce or better yet – stop caffeine, which is a stimulant that can trigger panic attacks and heart palpitations.

- Stop smoking – which "burns up" your nervous system.

- Unplug the phone and computer – for quiet time can help relieve stress. Write yourself a loving letter.

- Deep slow breathing exercises release tensions.

- Releasing your fears and overcoming self-doubt.

- Restful sleep and even daytime mini "cat" naps.

- Laughter – people who know how to laugh, smile and have fun are generally able to bounce back from stress.

- Don't be afraid to ask for help when you need it!

- Don't make impulsive snap judgements – take time.

- Realize that you can't change the past – learn from your past pain and let it serve your inner growth.

- You can't change others – you can only change yourself and your attitude. Be a strong, positive health captain.

Soothing Remedies for Tension Headaches

Ginger (*Zingiber officinale*) is helpful for tension headaches because it helps decrease the production of pain-causing prostaglandins. Also the simple pleasure of taking a break to make and drink a cup of herbal tea which will promote a feeling of relaxation and helps to relieve tension and stress. Also try combining ginger with chamomile, peppermint and linden blossom (mild relaxants). Have up to 4 cups daily. Here are the recipes for this ginger-herbal tea and other remedies for soothing tension. Relax and enjoy!

Ginger–Herbal Tea

Simmer 2 tsps fresh grated ginger or powered ginger in 2 cups distilled water in covered pan for 5 minutes. Add 2 tsps dried linden blossoms, 1 tsp each of dried chamomile and peppermint leaves. Cover and steep for 15 minutes. Then strain, sweeten with honey or the herb stevia if desired and enjoy (See page 177).

Linden-Flower Herbal Tea

To relieve nervous tension and promote relaxation, add 1 tsp of the following herb mixture to 1 cup boiling water; 2 oz linden-flowers, 1 oz sage, 1 oz thyme, 1 oz lemon balm. Steep 15 minutes and strain. Drink hour before bed.

Kava Herbal Remedy

The herb Kava, $^1/_2$ tsp of extract tincture in juice, will help relieve tension headaches in five minutes. Also helps relax the muscles in the neck and shoulders and relieves anxiety.

Headache Acupressure Points

Apply thumb pressure lightly on these pressure points.

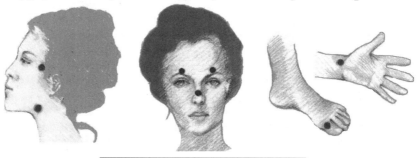

Peppermint Oil has been used for centuries for relief from nerve related issues. Peppermint helps suppress pain and is also used to fight mental fatigue and improve concentration. It has a cooling action on the skin and is used to relieve skin irritations and itchiness. – Dr. Bob Martin, *Secret Nerve Cures*

Scientists Reveal That Certain Foods Can Alter Your Mood

If you want to relieve stress naturally you may want to reach for carbohydrate-rich foods such as fresh fruits, vegetables, whole grain breads, cereals and pastas. These elevate serotonin levels which scientists have found help people feel more relaxed and calm. Judith Wurtman, a research scientist at the Massachusetts Institute of Technology's Brain and Cognitive Sciences Department, and author of *Managing Your Mind and Mood Through Food* says, *(amazon.com). "When people consume enough carbohydrates – between 35 to 40 grams – on an empty stomach, they will have the edge taken off their mood and feel better. Low serotonin levels are linked with increased aggression and depression."* Wurtman's research has also shown that high protein foods such as beans, nuts and soy products, release other substances that increase alertness and allow people to react and think more quickly. Studies done at the National Institutes of Health revealed that a diet containing omega-3 fat, is responsible for a decreased risk of depression, because it helps manipulate brain chemicals to boost mood. Omega-3 fats can be found in ground flaxseed, flax oil and walnuts.

SAMe: A Safe Natural Antidepressant

SAMe (S-adenosylmethionine), is an effective nutritional supplement that helps lift the clouds of depression and fortifies aching joints. According to a health article in *Newsweek (newsweek.com)*, in dozens of European trials that involved thousands of patients, SAMe has performed as well as traditional treatments for major depression and arthritis. Research also suggests SAMe can ease normally intractable liver conditions as well. SAMe hasn't shown adverse effects, and doctors have prescribed it successfully for two decades in the 14 countries where it has been approved as a drug. SAMe has been successfully used in Europe for over 20 years. SAMe's benefits were first reported in 1973 in Italy, where it is commonly recommended for depression. In one study, researchers found that SAMe worked as well as the prescription antidepressants like Elavil, Norpramin, Prozac and Sinequan without their toxic side effects. SAMe has been shown to increase levels of happy chemicals in the brain, such as serotonin and dopamine – without side effects such as agitation, nausea, insomnia and headaches, which are common in prescribed antidepressants (see web: *www.lef.org*).

In treating osteoarthritis, SAMe has proven beneficial and safe; 71% of a test group had very good results. SAMe was shown to be as effective and even better then Motrin, Advil, Naprosyn and Aleve. Studies also found that SAMe helps restore and maintain damaged cartilage. See website: *www.mothernature.com* for more info.

SAMe is a naturally occurring molecule found in virtually all body tissues and fluids. It acts as a methyl donor in biochemical reactions and is therefore involved in producing and processing a wide range of chemicals that maintain normal cell function. Since it is a naturally occurring substance, SAMe appears less likely to cause adverse side effects than synthesized drugs. Low levels of SAMe in your blood hinders the liver's efficiency to cleanse toxins from your body. SAMe supports and promotes the health of many body functions, including joint mobility and comfort, mood and emotional well-being.

St. John's Wort Relieves Depression

St. John's Wort was named for John the Baptist in the Bible, whose birthday, June 24, falls near the time this plant produces its flowers. The word *wort* means *plant* in Old English. St. John's Wort (*hypericum perforatum*), has been used in traditional herbal medicines for many centuries, primarily for wound healing. Recently, researchers believe this plant is also an SSRI – a class of antidepressant medication. A major study published in the *British Medical Journal,* (*depression.about.com*) showed that 55% of the 1,751 patients tested, had depression relief with St. John's Wort. The relief obtained was similar to that experienced from prescription antidepressants. St. John's Wort usually costs about $15 a month, considerably less than pharmaceutical antidepressants, and it does not cause the toxic side effects of other SSRIs. However, St. John's Wort sometimes may cause a dry mouth, some itching and a sensitive stomach. Don't take St. John's Wort when you are taking a pharmaceutical antidepressant.

St. John's Wort contains hypericin with anti-inflammatory properties and was used historically to relieve nerve pain especially resulting from injury, strain and shingles. Braggzyme Systemic Enzymes (see page 218) also has healing anti-inflammatory that acts in same way.

Enhance Mood and Mind with Vitamin B1

For decades, researchers have known vitamin B1 (*thiamine – often called the morale vitamin*) has a strong relationship to a healthy nervous system and mental attitude. To test the vitamin's mental status, researchers conducted a study of 120 female college students. The women were split into 2 groups, one taking 50 mg of B1 daily for 2 months and the other receiving a placebo. At study's end, researchers found B1 improved moods and also was safe and effective. Safe dosage of B1 is 50 to 100 mg. (Remember, natural supplements are the best.)

Help For Bipolar Disorder Mood Swings

Fish oil (omega-3) helps calm the volatile mood swings that are the hallmark of bipolar disorder – also known as manic depression. In a 4 month study of 30 people with bipolar disorder (*prevention.com*), those who took fish oil supplements in addition to their regular medication, saw greater improvement in symptoms than those who did not. Fish oil is rich in omega-3 fatty acids, which seem to tone down the over-active signaling between brain cells that may contribute to mood swings, according to medical researchers at the Baylor College of Medicine in Houston, Texas. See web: *www.bcm.edu/*

NADH: the coenzyme in the form of vitamin B3, niacin, helps convert the amino acid tyrosine into the important brain chemical dopamine. Dopamine is involved in mood, energy and sexual drive. According to Austrian researchers, NADH energizes both body and brain activity and improves alertness, concentration, emotions, drive and overall mood enhancement.

Vinpocetine: an Herbal Extract from the periwinkle plant, can dilate blood vessels, enhance circulation to the brain, make red blood cells more pliable, act as an antioxidant and inhibit aggregation of platelets. Researchers have found that vinpocetine appears to be beneficial in cognitive disorders that are due to poor blood flow to the brain. Individuals with atherosclerotic vascular disease may benefit from vinpocetine.

195

No man is free who is not master of himself. – Epictetus, 55-135 AD

Acetyl-L-Carnitine: helps in energy metabolism and the production of acetylcholine – a brain chemical involved in memory. It can remove toxic accumulations of fatty acids from the mitochondria, keeping these organelles healthy and functioning at their best; helps stabilize cell membranes and protect synapses and brain cells against damage from oxidation. Researchers in Milan, Italy, at the famous Mario Negri Institute for Pharmacological Research, found that acetyl-L-carnitine helped lower the rate of deterioration from Alzheimer's disease and age-related cognitive decline.

Huperzine-A: is an extract from club moss, and has inhibited acetylcholinesterase, the enzyme that breaks down acetylcholine in the brain. Alzheimer's disease is a condition in which there's a relative shortage of acetylcholine. Scientists at Zhejiang Medical University in China, have found that Alzheimer's patients treated with Huperzine-A had improvements in memory and other mental abilities. Other beneficial supplements are: Ginkgo Biloba, SAMe, St. John's Wort (pages 193-194, 197).

Foods Can Trigger Stress-Related Migraines

Researchers in London reported that after studying 88 children with severe migraines who had eliminated "trigger" foods from their diet, 78 of the children improved greatly. In adults, between 20 to 50% have a reduction of their headaches when trigger foods are avoided. Trigger foods have a reaction in the blood vessels and nerves which causes migraines. The trigger foods to avoid are: dairy products, chocolate, sugars, sodas, eggs and meat.

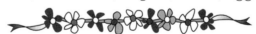

Avoid Health-Destroying Habits: Sugar, fat, salt, refined foods and refined flours, chemical preservatives, soda, soft drinks and alcohol.

Enthusiasm is one of the most powerful engines of success. When you do a thing, do it with all your might! Be active, be energetic, be enthusiastic and faithful, and you will accomplish your objective. – Ralph Waldo Emerson

---

The greatest mistake you can make in life is to be continually fearing a mistake you might never make. – Elbert Hubbard, 1885

Refusing to ask for help when needed, is refusing someone the chance to be helpful.

Ginkgo Biloba Helps Depression, Stroke and Brain Recovery

Ginkgo Biloba improves blood flow through the brain and aids in stroke recovery and mental acuity. It appears to normalize neurotransmitter levels and can help treat depression. In one European study, 80 mg of ginkgo biloba extract was given three times a day to a test group of 40 elderly individuals. After a few months, depression lifted and their mental faculties improved significantly. People taking blood thinners should probably avoid ginkgo until off the blood thinners.

Candida – A Fungus Linked to Chronic Fatigue, Bloating and Nausea

According to Joseph Pizzorno Jr., N.D., author of *Total Wellness, "Candida (a fungus) in some parts of the body such as the stomach and the vagina, can be relieved by lowering your intake of refined sugars. Sugar is the preferred food of fungi! Even those suffering from ulcers, have higher levels of fungi in their systems."* To improve your health and rid yourself of candida it is advised that you dramatically decrease the amount, or better yet, it's best to stop all refined carbohydrates – not only sugar and sweet products, but also white-flour products in your diet. Dr. Pizzorno says you can combat fungi naturally by taking the following:

197

Garlic: An anti-fungal agent; use 4 grams daily, or eat 1-2 cloves daily (mashed over salads, veggies, soups, etc.).

Caprylic Acid: Naturally occurring fatty acid that inhibits fungal growth; use: 1,000 mg with a meal.

Healthy Benefits from Eating Garlic

Ancient Egyptians and Romans prized the extraordinary healing powers of garlic. Garlic has potent immune-enhancing properties. It may eradicate many types of bacteria and fungi, including salmonella and candida, as well as inhibit gastrointestinal ulcers.

Garlic's papery skin should be peeled off and the hard roots trimmed at the end. After you chop garlic, let it sit for 10 minutes before cooking or eating, to let the beneficial enzymes develop.

The Fast Growing Healing Revolution: Alternative Health Therapies

According to new millennium studies reported in the *Journal of the American Medical Association*, nearly two-thirds of the nation's 125 traditional U.S. Medical Schools now teach alternative therapies including: massage, chiropractic, acupuncture, herbal medicine and mind-body medicine. Integrative medicine – a blending of complementary and alternative medicine – is the fastest growing segment of the healthcare industry. A study found 1 in 3 Americans had used alternative therapies, spending over 18 billion annually. This consumer-driven movement is now being joined by physicians who used to scoff at holistic medicine, and by many health insurers who previously had refused to pay for holistic therapies. *"The high-cost and purely scientific approach to medicine needs serious rethinking,"* said Dr. Samuel Benjamin, director Center for Complementary and Alternative Medicine, New York's Stonybrook School of Medicine.

"Complementary or Alternative Medicine is forcing U.S. healthcare to look at different approaches to healthcare, also achieving healthier communities."

The U.S. Congress agrees and has doubled its funds appropriated for the National Center for Complementary and Alternative Medicine, from $20 to $50 million. This is a positive step towards better health for Americans!

Control & Extend Your Health & Lifespan!

In the final analysis, it's up to you! No one can control your eating and living habits except yourself. You may take your troubles to experts, but all they can do is tell you what you should do. They can't do it for you. Most of your problems of living cannot be solved by someone else . . . only you! In this book we have given you the results of a lifetime of experience in the field of natural living and building a Powerful Nerve Force. This is all we can do. Now it's up to you to apply these teachings in your own life, to help solve your own problems and fill your own needs! Our prayers and love go with you daily as you strive to become more peaceful and healthy.

Paul C. Bragg and *Patricia Bragg*

Genesis 6:3 ~~~~~~~~~ 3 John 2

Chapter 15

Alternative Health Therapies And Massage Techniques

Try Them – They are Working Miracles for Millions!

Explore these wonderful natural methods of healing your body. Finally over 600 Medical Schools in the U.S. are teaching Healthy Alternative Therapies. Please check out the websites. Now seek and choose the best healing techniques for you:

ACUPUNCTURE/ACUPRESSURE: Acupuncture directs and rechannels body energy by inserting hair-thin needles (*use only disposable needles*) at specific points on the body. It's used for pain, backaches, migraines and general health and body dysfunctions. Used in Asia for centuries, acupuncture is safe, virtually painless and has no side effects. **Acupressure** is based on the same principles and uses finger pressure and massage rather than needles. Websites offer info, check them out: *acupuncturetoday.com* or *acupressure.com*

CHIROPRACTIC: was founded in Davenport, Iowa in 1885 by **199** Daniel David Palmer. There are now many schools in the U.S., and graduates are joining Health Practitioners in all nations of the world to share healing techniques. Chiropractic is popular and the largest U.S. healing profession benefitting literally millions! Treatment involves soft tissue, spinal and body adjustment to free the nervous system of interferences with normal body function. Its concern is the functional integrity of the musculoskeletal system. In addition to manual methods, chiropractors use physical therapy modalities, exercise, health and nutritional guidance. Web: *chiroweb.com*

F. MATHIUS ALEXANDER TECHNIQUE: These lessons help end improper use of neuromuscular system and bring body posture back into balance. Eliminates psycho-physical interferences, helps release long-held tension, and aids in re-establishing muscle tone. Web: *www.alexandertechnique.com*

FELDENKRAIS METHOD: Dr. Moshe Feldenkrais founded this in the late 1940s. This Method leads to improved posture and helps create ease and more efficiency of body movement. This Method is a great stress removal. Web: *feldenkrais.com*

Physical Therapy & Massage helps promote healing & helps with respiratory, nervous disorders, asthma, emphysema, etc. It helps relieve pain, improve blood flow, correct posture & promote health. – Dr. Linda Page, Author of *Healthy Healing*

Alternative Health Therapies & Massage Techniques

HOMEOPATHY: In the 1800's, Dr. Samuel Hahnemann developed homeopathy. Patients are treated with "micro" doses of remedies found in nature to trigger the body's own defenses. This homeopathic principle is a safe and nontoxic remedy and is the #1 alternative therapy in Europe and Britain because it is inexpensive, seldom has any side effects, and usually brings fast results. Web: *www.homeopathic.org*

NATUROPATHY: Brought to America by Dr. Benedict Lust, M.D., this treatment uses diet, herbs, homeopathy, fasting, exercise, hydrotherapy, manipulation and sunlight. (Dr. Paul C. Bragg graduated from Dr. Lust's first School of Naturopathy in the U.S. Now 6 schools) Practitioners work with your body to restore health naturally. They reject surgery and drugs except as a last resort. Web: *www.naturopathic.org*

OSTEOPATHY: The first School of Osteopathy was founded in 1892 by Dr. Andrew Taylor Still, M.D. There are now 15 U.S. colleges. Treatment involves soft tissue, spinal and body adjustments that free the nervous system from interferences that can cause illness. Healing by adjustment also includes good nutrition, physical therapies, proper breathing and good posture. Dr. Still's premise: if the body structure is altered or abnormal, then proper body function is altered and can cause pain and illness. Web: *www.osteopathic.org*

REFLEXOLOGY OR ZONE THERAPY: Founded by Eunice Ingham, author of *Stories The Feet Can Tell*, inspired by a Bragg Health Crusade when she was 17. Reflexology helps the body and organs by removing crystalline deposits from reflex areas (nerve endings) of feet and hands through deep pressure massage. Primitive reflexology originated in China and Egypt and Native American Indians and Kenyans self-practiced it for centuries. Reflexology activates the body's flow of healing and energy by dislodging deposits. Visit Eunice Ingham and nephew Dwight Byer's web: *www.reflexology-usa.net*

SKIN BRUSHING: – Daily is wonderful for circulation, toning, cleansing and healing. Use a dry vegetable brush (never nylon) and brush lightly. Helps purify lymph so it's able to detoxify your blood and tissues. Removes old skin cells, uric acid crystals and toxic wastes that come up through skin's pores. Use loofah sponge for variety in shower or tub.

"Homeopathy *cures a larger percentage of cases than most any other method of treatment and is beyond a doubt safer and has proven to be the most complete medical science."* – Mahatma Gandhi

Alternative Health Therapies & Massage Techniques

REIKI: A Japanese form of massage that means "Universal Life Energy." The Reiki Massage helps the body to detoxify, then re-balance and heal itself. Discovered in the ancient Sutra manuscripts by Dr. Mikao Usui in 1822. Web: *www.reiki.org*

ROLFING: Developed by Ida Rolf in the 1930's in the U.S. Rolfing is also called structural processing and postural release, or structural dynamics. It is based on the concept that distortions (accidents, injuries, falls, etc.) and the effects of gravity on the body cause upsets and long-term stress in the body. Rolfing helps to achieve balance and improved body posture. Methods involve the use of stretching, gentle deep tissue massage and relaxation techniques to loosen old injuries, break bad movement and posture patterns. Web: *rolf.org*

TRAGERING: Founded by Dr. Milton Trager M.D., who was inspired at age 18 by Paul C. Bragg to become a doctor. It is a mind-body learning method that involves gentle shaking and rocking, allowing the body to let go, releasing tensions and lengthening the muscles for more body peace and health. Tragering can do miracle healing where needed in the body frame, muscles and the entire body. Web: *trager.com*

WATER THERAPY: Soothing detox shower: apply Bragg Olive Oil to skin, alternate hot and cold water, every 2-3 minutes. Massage body while under hot, filtered spray. Garden hose massage is great in summer or anytime. Hot detox soak bath (diabetics use warm water) 20 minutes with cup of Epsom salts or apple cider vinegar. This soak helps pull out the toxins by creating an artificial fever cleanse. Web: *holisticonline.com/hydrotherapy.htm*

MASSAGE & AROMATHERAPY: – Works two ways: the essence (aroma) relaxes, as does healing massages. Essential oils are extracted from flowers, leaves, roots, seeds and barks. These are usually massaged into the skin, inhaled or used in a bath for their ability to relax, soothe and heal. The oils, used for centuries to treat numerous ailments, are revitalizing and energizing for the body and mind. Example: Tiger balm, MSM, echinacea and arnica help relieve muscle aches. (Avoid skin creams and lotions with mineral oil – it clogs the skin's pores.) Use these natural oils for the skin: almond, apricot kernel, avocado, and I use Bragg Organic Olive Oil and mix with aromatic essential oils: rosemary, lavender, rose, jasmine, sandalwood or lemon-balm, etc. – 6 oz. oil and 4 drops of an essential oil. Web: *naha.org*

Alternative Health Therapies & Massage Techniques

MASSAGE – SELF: Paul C. Bragg often said, "You can be your own best massage therapist, even if you have only one good hand." Near-miraculous health improvements have been achieved by victims of accidents or strokes in bringing life back to afflicted parts of their own bodies by self-massage and even vibrators. Treatments can be day or night, almost continual. Self-massage also helps achieve relaxation at day's end. Families and friends can learn and exchange massages; it's a wonderful sharing experience. Remember, babies love and thrive with their daily massages, start from birth. Family pets also love their soothing, healing touch of massages. Web: *rd.com/health/learn-the-art-of-self-massage*.

MASSAGE – SHIATSU: Japanese form of health massage that applies pressure from the fingers, hands, elbows and even knees along the same points as acupuncture. Shiatsu has been used in Asia for centuries to relieve pain, common ills, muscle stress and to aid lymphatic circulation. Web: *shiatsu.org*

202

MASSAGE – SPORTS: An important health support system for professional and amateur athletes. Sports massage improves circulation and mobility to injured tissue, enables athletes to recover more rapidly from myofascial injury, reduces muscle soreness and chronic strain patterns. Soft tissues are freed of trigger points and adhesions, thus contributing to improvement of peak neuro-muscular functioning and athletic performance.

MASSAGE – SWEDISH: One of the oldest and the most popular and widely used massage techniques. This deep body massage soothes and promotes healthy circulation and is a great way to loosen and relax tight muscles before and after exercise. See web: *www.massageden.com/swedish-massage.shtml*

Author's Comments: We have personally sampled many of these Alternative Therapies. It's estimated that soon America's health care costs will leap to over 2 trillion. It's more important than ever to be responsible for our own health! This includes seeking holistic health practitioners who are dedicated to keeping us well by inspiring us to practice prevention! These Alternative Healing Therapies are also popular and getting results: aroma, Ayurvedic, biofeedback, color, guided imagery, herbs, music, meditation, magnets, saunas, tai chi, chi gong, Pilates, Rebounder, yoga, etc. Explore them and be open to improving your earthly temple for a healthy, happier, longer life. **Seek & find the best for your body, mind & soul. – Patricia Bragg, ND, PhD.**

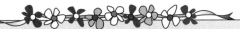

Our Personal Health Message to You

You can become a powerhouse of dynamic energy and vitality. You can build an inexhaustible reservoir of powerful Nerve Force. Nothing can stop you except yourself.

Remember Life Flows Through Your Nerves and that you alone have the power to generate the needed Nerve Force which is going to flow through your nerves. But you must work and earn it! It won't be handed to you on a silver platter. You must earn the good things of life. Everything in life has a price tag. What you put into this Nerve Force Building Program is what you will reap from it – no more, no less – it's all up to you!

There is absolutely nothing complicated about the Program that we have outlined for you in this book. It is a simple, natural healthy lifestyle. Follow it and you can become a human dynamo regardless of your age.

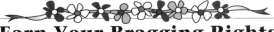

Earn Your Bragging Rights
Live The Bragg Healthy Lifestyle
To Attain Supreme Physical,
Mental, Emotional and Spiritual Health!

203

God bless you and your family and may He give you the strength, the courage and the patience to win your battle to re-enter the Healthy Garden of Eden while you are still living here on Earth with time to enjoy it all!!!

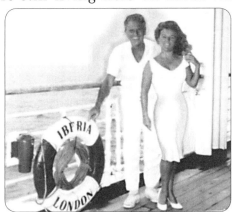

Health Crusaders Paul Bragg and daughter Patricia traveled the world spreading health, inspiring millions to renew and revitalize their health and life.

3 John 2 is the Bragg Crusade

We have love for you and God loves you –
pass it along and share this wisdom and love,

Paul and *Patricia*

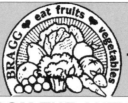

FROM THE AUTHORS

This book was written for You! It can be your passport to a healthy, long, vital life. We in the Alternative Health Therapies join hands in one common objective – promoting a high standard of health for everyone. Healthy nutrition points the way – which is Mother Nature and God's Way. This book teaches you how to work with them, not against them! Health Doctors, therapists nurses, teachers and caregivers are becoming more dedicated than ever before to keeping their patients healthy and fit. This book was written to emphasize the great needed importance of healthy lifestyle living for health and longevity, close to Mother Nature and God.

Statements in this book are scientific health findings, known facts of physiology and biological therapeutics. Paul C. Bragg practiced natural methods of living for over 80 years with highly beneficial results, knowing that they were safe and of great value. His daughter Patricia lectured and co-authored the Bragg Health Books with him and continues to carrying on The Bragg Health Crusades.

204

Paul C. Bragg and daughter Patricia express their opinions solely as Public Health Educators and Health Crusaders. They offer no cure for disease. Only the body has the ability to cure a person. Experts may disagree with some of the statements made in this book. However, such statements are considered to be factual, based on the long-time experience of dedicated pioneer health crusaders Paul C. Bragg and Patricia Bragg. If you suspect you have a medical problem, please seek qualified health care professionals to help you make the healthiest, wisest and best-informed choices!

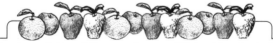

Count your blessings daily while you do your 30 to 45 minute brisk walks and exercises with these affirmations – health! strength! youth! vitality! peace! laughter! humility! understanding! forgiveness! joy! and love for eternity! – and soon all these qualities will come flooding and bouncing into your life. With blessings of super health, peace and love to you, our dear friends – our readers. – Patricia Bragg

If I were to name the three most precious resources of life, I would say books, friends and nature; and the greatest of these, at least the most constant and always at hand is Mother Nature and God. – John Burroughs

Change your lifestyle to healthy living, then you will improve your life!

Everything in excess is opposed by nature. – Hippocrates, Father of Medicine

BRAGG Build Powerful Nerve Force

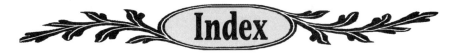

Index

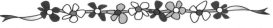

Touch is a primal need, as necessary for growth as food, clothing or shelter. Michelangelo knew this when he painted God extending a hand toward Adam on ceiling of Sistine Chapel, he chose touch to depict the gift of life. – George H. Colt

When you sell a man a book you don't just sell him paper, ink and glue, you sell him a whole new life! There's heaven and earth in a real book, and the main purpose of books is to trap the mind into its own thinking and action.
– Christopher Morley

INDEX

C

Cabbage, 43, 72, 88-89, 93, 97, 105, 112-115

Caffeine (coffee), 9, 19, 21, 26, 39, 41, 44-45, 47, 67, 71-72, 77-78, 80, 85-86, 101, 109, 159, 161, 163, 172, 174, 185, 191

Calcium, 33, 60, 71, 77, 83-84, 89, 91-95, 102, 128, 158-159, 172, 175, 182-185, 187-188, 190

Cancer, 18, 32, 41, 47, 84, 95, 97-98, 111, 113, 121, 127-128, 136, 143-145, 147, 169, 173, 185, 188-189

Candida, 34, 174, 197

Capillaries, 65, 80-81, 84, 86, 97

Carbohydrates, 102, 119, 187, 193, 197

Cardiovascular Disease, 35, 42, 87-88, 184, 188

Cataracts, 128, 136

Cayenne (capsaicin), 89, 114, 128, 182

Chelation, 183-184

Children, 5, 14-15, 17, 19, 30, 33, 48, 67, 81, 91-92, 94, 111, 117-118, 128, 131, 133, 136, 150, 153, 157, 169-172, 176-177, 179, 196

Chiropractic, 128, 163, 173, 199

Chlorine, 140, 143-145

Cholesterol, 17, 31-33, 56, 84, 94, 97, 101, 103, 116, 127-128, 143-145, 159, 183, 185

Chondroitin, 128

Chronic Fatigue (CFS), 13, 170, 172-175, 197

Circulation, 12, 26-27, 35, 46, 59, 68-69, 108, 120-121, 127, 132, 140, 152, 195, 200, 202

Cleansing, 7, 15, 96, 108, 116, 135, 139, 200

Constipation, 12, 42-43, 46, 75, 133, 162

D

Depression, 2-3, 15, 22, 30-31, 42, 74-75, 87, 94, 118-119, 127, 153, 156, 173, 179, 182, 185, 188-190, 193-195, 197

Detoxification, 97, 104, 108

Diabetes, 3, 17, 32-33, 42, 84, 87, 100, 111, 121, 127, 136, 147, 175

Diet, 17, 19, 21, 23, 26, 32-33, 39, 41-43, 67, 71, 81-116, 128, 158, 169, 171-182, 189, 193, 196-197, 200

Digestion, 7, 12, 40-41, 43-44, 46, 72, 100, 104, 108, 128, 133, 151

Distilled Water, 18, 26, 43, 83, 106-108, 128, 146, 174

Drugs, 9-10, 14, 35, 39, 41, 45, 47, 78, 80-81, 86, 101, 103, 136, 152, 159, 163, 170-171, 185, 189-190, 194, 200

E

Elimination, 108-109, 116, 128, 133, 139

Emphysema, 136, 164, 199

Energy, 3, 5, 10, 20-21, 26, 29-30, 32, 36, 38-39, 42-44, 46, 49-53, 58, 63, 65-66, 68, 73, 79, 86-87, 102, 104, 108-109, 117, 120, 127, 146, 150, 155, 160, 164, 170, 174, 177, 187, 191, 195-196, 199-201, 203

Essential Fatty Acids, 83, 98, 196-197

Exercise, 6, 16, 22, 26-27, 32-33, 42, 45, 58, 60, 67, 69-72, 77, 80, 87, 95, 117-128, 131, 140, 142, 146, 148, 150, 153, 156, 162-163, 165, 171, 173, 175, 179, 189, 191, 199-200, 202, 204

Eyes, 59, 78, 96, 109, 135, 145, 185

When you can think of yesterday without regret, and of tomorrow without fear, then you are on the road to success.

Follow the steps of the godly instead, and stay on the right path, for good men enjoy life to the full. – Proverbs 2:20-21

Live a balanced life – learn some and think some and draw and paint and sing and dance and play and work some every day.
– Robert Fulghum, author, *All I Really Need to Know I Learned in Kindergarten*

Good health, generated by physical fitness is the logical starting point for the pursuit of excellence in any field. Physical vitality promotes mental vitality and thus is essential to executive achievement.
– Dr. Richard E. Dutton, University of Southern Florida

I expect to pass through this life but once. Therefore, if there be any kindness I can show, or any good deed I can do, let me do it now and not defer or neglect it! – William Penn, English Philosopher, 1644-1718

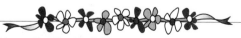

Your Daily Habits Form Your Future

Habits can be wrong, good or bad, healthy or unhealthy, rewarding or unrewarding. The right or wrong habits, decisions, actions, words or deeds . . . are up to you! Wisely choose your habits, as they can make or break your life! – Patricia Bragg

INDEX

All our dreams can come true – if we have the courage to pursue them.
– Walt Disney, famous creator Disneyland, Disney movies

I am beginning to learn that it is the sweet, simple things of life which are the real ones after all. – Laura Ingalls Wilder, Author

A gift is pure when it is given from the heart to the right person at the right time and at the right place and when we expect nothing in return.

INDEX

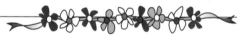

*Your life will improve, glow and
sparkle with health,
if you allow it to!!!*

HOW?

*If you will take charge, then guide and
control your life with health wisdom and
love – then you can reach your health goals!!!
With love and prayers to you – our health friends.*

– Patricia Bragg, N.D., Ph.D., Health Crusader

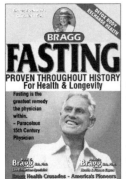
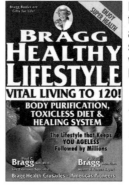
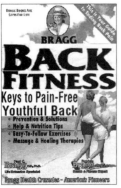
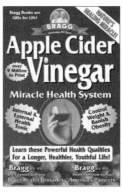
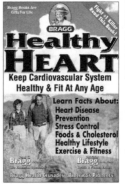
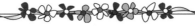

BRAGG HEALTH BOOKS
ARE GIFTS FOR LIFE

Gen. 6:3 | 3 John 2

– Jack LaLanne, Bragg follower since 15 years old

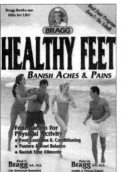

Learn how to banish aches & pains. Read about Reflexology, Acupressure and much more. Almost all of us are born with perfect feet. It's the abuse millions give their feet that makes them cry as they limp through life - "my aching feet are killing me!" Read this book!

The Bragg Foot Program is the best. I thank Bragg Books and their wisdom for my long, active, healthy life.
– Dr. Scholl,
Famous Foot Doctor

978-0-87790-077-1 – $9.95

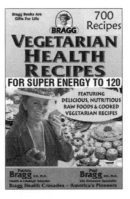

Enjoy the worlds finest health recipes for super health and high energy that you and your family will love. Over 700 Healthy Recipes for Health, Super Energy and Longevity. 336 pages filled with delicious raw and cooked foods, vegan and vegetarian recipes.

This book shows how to eat right with nutritious recipes to maintain your body's health and fitness.
– Henry Hoegerman, M.D.

978-0-87790-027-6 – $13.95

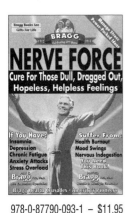

Millions of healthy, happy followers have learned to control and increase their Vital Nerve Force Energy - The Bragg Healthy Way. Here's Prevention and Health Maintenance all in one book.

I have my life back after many years of chronic fatigue, fibromyalgia and clinical depression. I give thanks to The Bragg Health Books.
– Marilyn Mason

978-0-87790-093-1 – $11.95

Breathing deeply, fully and completely energizes, calms, fills you with peace and keeps you youthful. Learn Bragg Breathing Exercises for more go-power and Super Health!

Thanks to Paul Bragg and Bragg Books, my years of asthma were cured in only one month with The Bragg Super Breathing and Bragg Healthy Lifestyle Living!
– Paul Wenner,
Gardenburger Creator

978-0-87790-120-4 – $11.95

"I thank Paul Bragg and the Bragg Healthy Lifestyle for my healthy, long, active life. I love Bragg Books and Health Products."
– Jack LaLanne, Bragg follower to 96½ years young

I have followed "The Bragg Healthy Lifestyle for years and it teaches you to take control of your health and build a healthy future."
– Mark Victor Hansen, Co-Producer, *Chicken Soup for the Soul* Series

"Thanks to Bragg Books for my conversion to the healthy way."
– James F. Balch, M.D.,
Co-Author of – *Prescription for Nutritional Healing*

"Bragg Books have been a blessing to our family and the TBN family of loyal viewers."
– Evangelist Dwight Thompson – *Co-Host TBN "Praise The Lord"*

If Bragg Books are unavailable in your area you may order:
on-line at: www.bragg.com or see Bragg book list.
Bragg Book Special: All 10 books for only $89 Postpaid.

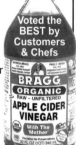

BRAGG ORGANIC APPLE CIDER VINEGAR

SIZE	PRICE	UPS SHIPPING & HANDLING For USA	$ Amount
16 oz.	$ 3.49 each	S/H – Please add $9. for 1st bottle and $1.50 each additional bottle	•
16 oz.	$ 38.00 Special Case /12	S/H Cost by Time Zone: CA $12. PST/MST $14. CST $22. EST $25	•
32 oz.	$ 5.59 each	S/H – Please add $10. for 1st bottle – $2. each additional bottle	•
32 oz.	$ 61.00 Special Case /12	S/H Cost by Time Zone: CA $17. PST/MST $20. CST $35. EST $38	•
1 gal.	$ 17.49 each	S/H – 1st bottle: CA $10. PST/MST $10. CST $13. EST $15 – $6. each add'l bottle	•
1 gal.	$ 61.00 Special Case /4	S/H Cost by Time Zone: CA $17. PST/MST $20. CST $34. EST $37	•

BRAGG Vinegar is a food and not taxable	**BRAGG VINEGAR**	$	•
	(S&H) Shipping & Handling		•
	TOTAL	$	•

BRAGG LIQUID AMINOS

SIZE	PRICE	UPS SHIPPING & HANDLING For USA	$ Amount
6 oz.	$ 3.79 each	S/H – Please add $9. for 1st 3 bottles – $1.50 each additional bottle	•
6 oz.	$ 83.00 Special Case /24	S/H Cost by Time Zone: CA $10. PST/MST $11. CST $17. EST $19	•
16 oz.	$ 4.99 each	S/H – Please add $9. for 1st bottle – $1.50 each additional bottle	•
16 oz.	$ 54.00 Special Case /12	S/H Cost by Time Zone: CA $12. PST/MST $14. CST $22. EST $25	•
32 oz.	$ 8.19 each	S/H – Please add $9. for 1st bottle and $2. each additional bottle	•
32 oz.	$ 90.00 Special Case /12	S/H Cost by Time Zone: CA $17. PST/MST $20. CST $35. EST $38	•
1 gal.	$ 29.99 each	S/H – 1st bottle: CA $10. PST/MST $10. CST $13. EST $15 – $6. each add'l bottle	•
1 gal.	$ 104.00 Special Case /4	S/H Cost by Time Zone: CA $17. PST/MST $20. CST $34. EST $37	•

BRAGG Aminos & Olive Oil are foods and not taxable	**BRAGG AMINOS**	$	•
	(S&H) Shipping & Handling		•
	TOTAL	$	•

BRAGG ORGANIC OLIVE OIL

SIZE	PRICE	UPS SHIPPING & HANDLING For USA	$ Amount
16 oz.	$ 11.99 each	S/H – Please add $9. for 1st bottle – $1.50 each additional bottle	•
16 oz.	$ 131.00 Special Case /12	S/H Cost by Time Zone: CA $12. PST/MST $14. CST $22. EST $25	•
32 oz.	$ 19.49 each	S/H – Please add $10. for 1st bottle and $2. each additional bottle	•
32 oz.	$ 214.00 Special Case /12	S/H Cost by Time Zone: CA $17. PST/MST $20. CST $35. EST $38	•
1 gal.	$ 68.39 each	S/H – 1st bottle: CA $10. PST/MST $10. CST $13. EST $15 – $6. each add'l bottle	•
1 gal.	$ 239.00 Special Case /4	S/H Cost by Time Zone: CA $17. PST/MST $20. CST $34. EST $37	•

Please Specify: ☐ Check ☐ Money Order ☐ Cash	**BRAGG OLIVE OIL**	$	•
Charge to: ☐ Visa ☐ Master Card ☐ Discover	**(S&H) Shipping & Handling**		•

Credit Card Number:_____ Card Expires: ____ / ____ month / year

	TOTAL	$	•

VISA
MasterCard
DISCOVER

Signature:_____

Business office calls (805) 968-1020. We accept MasterCard, Discover & VISA phone orders. Please prepare order using order form. It speeds your call and serves as order record. Hours: 8 to 4 pm Pacific Time, Monday thru Friday.

• Visit our Web: www.bragg.com • e-mail: bragg @ bragg.com

CREDIT CARD ORDERS
CALL **(800) 446-1990**
8 am-4 pm PST • Mon.-Fri.
OR FAX **(805) 968-1001**

Mail to: **HEALTH SCIENCE, Box 7, Santa Barbara, CA 93102 USA** BOF 1011
Please Print or Type – Be sure to give street & house number to facilitate delivery.

• **Name**

• **Address** **Apt. No.**

• **City** **State** **Zip**

• ( ) **Phone** **e-mail**

Bragg Health Products available most Health Stores & Grocery Health Depts Nationwide

BRAGG HEALTHY SALAD DRESSINGS

ORGANIC HEALTHY VINAIGRETTE

This Bragg Healthy Organic Vinaigrette Dressing makes a salad special with its tasty, tangy flavor. A zesty blend of Bragg Organic Extra Virgin Olive Oil, Bragg Organic Apple Cider Vinegar, Bragg Liquid Aminos, garlic, and onion, raw honey and delicious organic herbs. This unique taste brings you a healthy salad dressing for all your salads & vegetables. Bragg's is the healthy choice!

12 oz glass bottle

Made with Organic GINGER & SESAME

This Bragg Healthy Dressing is based on the delicious flavors of our famous Bragg Liquid Aminos and ginger's sweet and tangy taste. Great on salads and veggies, brings you the best of Bragg tradition – healthy eating and living.

12 oz glass bottle

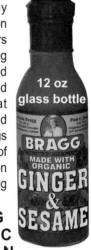

BRAGGBERRY ORGANIC Dressing & Marinade

Brings new taste treats, with Blueberries, Raspberries, Acai, Goji and Grape. Low-fat and natural antioxidants. All the best of Bragg's healthy tradition.

NEW

12 oz glass bottle

12 oz glass bottle

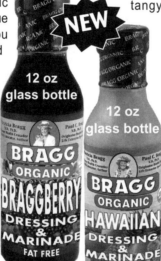

BRAGG ORGANIC HAWAIIAN Dressing & Marinade

Brings Taste of Aloha to salads, veggies, stir-frys and other healthy foods. Unlock Hawaiian secret flavors you will love with Bragg Natural Delicious and Tasty Hawaiian Dressing and Marinade.

America's Healthiest All-Purpose Seasonings

BRAGG SPRINKLE
ORGANIC 24 HERBS & SPICES

This old favorite is now available again. Bragg Sprinkle was created in 1931 by Paul C. Bragg, Health Pioneer & Originator Health Food Stores. Organic Sprinkle adds new healthy, delicious flavors to most recipes & meals. It's salt-free with no additives, preservatives or fillers.

SHAKER TOP

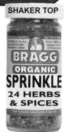

BRAGG ORGANIC KELP SEASONING

SHAKER TOP

This original Organic Kelp Seasoning made from sun-dried Organic Pacific Ocean Sea Kelp, combined with 24 all natural herbs and spices. It's a healthy, delicious seasoning for almost all recipes and meals and is specially suited for low-sodium diets.

NEW BRAGG Delicious Nutritional Yeast Seasoning

Nutritionally designed to help meet nutritional needs of vegetarians, vegans and anyone wanting a good source of B12, B-Complex Vitamins. It's "cheese-like" flavor makes it a delicious, healthy topping & seasoning.

SHAKER TOP

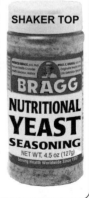

- Gluten-Free • Non-GMO
- No Salt • No Sugar • No Dairy
- No Artificial Colors & Preservatives
- No Brewery Products
- No Candida Albicans
- Vegetarian & Kosher Certified

You are what you eat, drink, breathe, think, say & do. – Patricia Bragg, ND, PhD.

BRAGG SPRINKLE – 24 Herbs & Spices Seasoning

SIZE	PRICE		UPS SHIPPING & HANDLING For USA	$	Amount
1.5 oz.	$ 4.99	each	S/H – Please add $9. for 1st 3 bottles and $1. each additional bottle		.
1.5 oz.	$ 54.00	Special Case /12	S/H Cost by Time Zone: CA $9. PST/MST $9. CST $10. EST $12.		.
BRAGG Sprinkle Seasoning is a food and not taxable			BRAGG SPRINKLE	$	.
			(S&H) Shipping & Handling		.
			TOTAL	$	.

BRAGG ORGANIC SEA KELP

2.7 oz.	$ 4.99	each	S/H – Please add $9. for 1st 3 bottles and $1. each additional bottle		.
2.7 oz.	$ 54.00	Special Case /12	S/H Cost by Time Zone: CA $9. PST/MST $9. CST $10. EST $12.		.
BRAGG Kelp Seasoning is a food and not taxable			BRAGG KELP	$	.
			(S&H) Shipping & Handling		.
			TOTAL	$	.

BRAGG NUTRITIONAL YEAST

4.5 oz.	$ 6.69	each	S/H – Please add $9. for 1st 3 bottles and $1. each additional bottle		.
4.5 oz.	$ 73.00	Special Case /12	S/H Cost by Time Zone: CA $9. PST/MST $9. CST $10. EST $12.		.
BRAGG Nutritional Yeast Seasoning is a food and not taxable			BRAGG YEAST	$	.
			(S&H) Shipping & Handling		.
			TOTAL	$	.

BRAGG SALAD DRESSINGS

✲ BRAGG GINGER & SESAME SALAD DRESSING

12 oz.	$ 5.79	each	S/H – Please add $9. for 1st bottle and $1.25 each additional bottle		.
12 oz.	$ 63.00	Special Case /12	S/H Cost by Time Zone: CA $11. PST/MST $12. CST $19. EST $22		.

✲ BRAGG ORGANIC VINAIGRETTE SALAD DRESSING

12 oz.	$ 5.79	each	S/H – Please add $9. for 1st bottle and $1.25 each additional bottle		.
12 oz.	$ 63.00	Special Case /12	S/H Cost by Time Zone: CA $11. PST/MST $12. CST $19. EST $22		.

✲ BRAGG BRAGGBERRY DRESSING & MARINADE

12 oz.	$ 5.79	each	S/H – Please add $9. for 1st bottle and $1.25 each additional bottle		.
12 oz.	$ 63.00	Special Case /12	S/H Cost by Time Zone: CA $11. PST/MST $12. CST $19. EST $22		.

✲ BRAGG HAWAIIAN DRESSING & MARINADE

12 oz.	$ 5.79	each	S/H – Please add $9. for 1st bottle and $1.25 each additional bottle		.
12 oz.	$ 63.00	Special Case /12	S/H Cost by Time Zone: CA $11. PST/MST $12. CST $19. EST $22		.
BRAGG Salad Dressings/Marinades are foods and not taxable			BRAGG SALAD DRESSINGS	$	.
			(S&H) Shipping & Handling		.
			TOTAL	$	.

Payment Method:

☐ Check ☐ Money Order ☐ Cash **Charge To:** ☐ Visa ☐ Master Card ☐ Discover

Credit Card Number:_____

Card Expires:_____ / _____
month / year

Signature:_____

VISA
MasterCard
DISCOVER

Business office calls (805) 968-1020. We accept MasterCard, Discover & VISA phone orders. Please prepare order using order form. It speeds your call and serves as order record. Hours: 8 to 4 pm Pacific Time, Monday thru Friday.
• Visit our Web: www.bragg.com • e-mail: bragg @ bragg.com

CREDIT CARD ORDERS
CALL **(800) 446-1990**
8 am - 4 pm PST • Mon.- Fri.
OR FAX **(805) 968-1001**

Mail to: **HEALTH SCIENCE, Box 7, Santa Barbara, CA 93102 USA**   BOF 1011
Please Print or Type – Be sure to give street & house number to facilitate delivery.

Name _____

Address _____ Apt. No. _____

City _____ State _____ Zip _____

(_____) _____
Phone   e-mail _____

Bragg Products available most Health Stores & Grocery Health Depts Nationwide

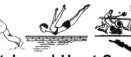

BRAGG ORGANIC APPLE CIDER VINEGAR DRINKS

FLAVORS	SIZE	PRICE	QTY	CASE/12 PRICE	QTY	$ Amount
Original Apple Cider Vinegar & Honey - 16 oz	$2.29			$25.00		.
ACV with Ginger - Spice - 16 oz	$2.29			$25.00		.
ACV with Apple - Cinnamon - 16 oz	$2.29			$25.00		.
ACV with Concord Grape - Acai - 16 oz	$2.29			$25.00		.
Apple Cider Vinegar & Sweet Stevia - 16 oz	$2.29			$25.00		.
Apple Cider Vinegar Limeade - 16 oz	$2.29			$25.00		.

BRAGG ORGANIC APPLE CIDER VINEGAR DRINKS are Foods and are not taxable

BRAGG VINEGAR DRINK	$	.
(S&H) Shipping & Handling		.

SHIPPING CHART FOR VINEGAR DRINKS

number of bottles	CA	PST/MST	CST	EST
1-2 bottles	$8.00	$8.00	$9.00	$12.00
3-4 bottles	$8.00	$9.00	$11.00	$13.00
5-6 bottles	$9.00	$9.00	$13.00	$15.00
7-12 bottles	$11.00	$13.00	$21.00	$24.00
Special Case/12	$11.00	$13.00	$21.00	$24.00

TOTAL $.

Please call around to Health & Grocery Stores first, because many now sell Bragg Health Products.

BRAGGZYME – Systemic Enzymes with CoQ10

SIZE	PRICE	UPS SHIPPING & HANDLING For USA	$ Amount
120 cap	$ 43.95 each	S/H – Please add $9. for 1st 3 bottles and $1. each additional bottle	.
120 cap	$ 483.00 Special Case /12	S/H Cost by Time Zone: CA $9. PST/MST $10. CST $11. EST $12.	.

on Braggzyme CA Residents only pay tax

for BRAGGZYME only CA Residents add 7.75% TAX	$	.
(S&H) Shipping & Handling		.

TOTAL $.

Payment Method:

☐ Check ☐ Money Order ☐ Cash

Charge To: ☐ Visa ☐ Master Card ☐ Discover

Credit Card Number:_____

Card Expires:_____ / _____
month / year

Signature:_____

We accept

VISA
MasterCard
DISCOVER

Business office calls (805) 968-1020

Phone orders please prepare order using order forms, as it speeds up your call and serves as your order record.

Hours: 8 to 4 pm Pacific Time, Monday thru Friday.

• Visit Web: www.bragg.com • e-mail: bragg @ bragg.com

CREDIT CARD ORDERS
CALL **(800) 446-1990**
8 am - 4 pm PST • Mon.- Fri.
OR FAX **(805) 968-1001**

BOF 1011

Mail to: **HEALTH SCIENCE, Box 7, Santa Barbara, CA 93102 USA**
Please Print or Type – Be sure to give street & house number to facilitate delivery.

_____
Name

_____
Address   **Apt. No.**

_____
City   **State**   **Zip**

(   )_____
Phone   **e-mail**

Bragg Products available most Health Stores & Grocery Health Depts Nationwide

Send for Free Health Bulletins

Patricia wants to keep in touch with you, your relatives and friends about the latest Health, Nutrition and Longevity Discoveries. Please enclose one stamp for each USA name listed or visit *www.bragg.com* and sign up for free health literature.

   With Blessings of Health, Peace and Thanks

Please make copy, then print clearly and mail to:

BRAGG HEALTH CRUSADES, Box 7, Santa Barbara, CA 93102

Name

Address   Apt. No.

City   State   Zip

Phone (   )   e-mail

Name

Address   Apt. No.

City   State   Zip

Phone (   )   e-mail

Name

Address   Apt. No.

City   State   Zip

Phone (   )   e-mail

Name

Address   Apt. No.

City   State   Zip

Phone (   )   e-mail

Name

Address   Apt. No.

City   State   Zip

Phone (   )   e-mail

Bragg Health Crusades spreading health worldwide since 1912

PATRICIA BRAGG, N.D., Ph.D.
Health Crusader & Angel of Health & Healing

Author, Lecturer, Nutritionist, Health & Lifestyle Educator to World Leaders, Hollywood Stars, Singers, Athletes, etc. & Millions

Patricia is a 100% Health Crusader with a lifetime dedication passion like her father, Paul C. Bragg, world renowned health authority. Patricia has won international fame on her own. She conducts Bragg Health & Fitness Seminars & Lectures for Conventions & Schools, Women's, Men's, Youth & Church Groups world-wide. She promotes Bragg Healthy Lifestyle Living & "How-To, Self-Health" Books on Radio & TV Talk Shows throughout the English-speaking world. Consultants to Presidents & Royalty, to Stars of Stage, Screen & TV & to Champion Athletes, Patricia & her Father co-authored The Bragg Health Library of Instructive, Inspiring Books that promote a healthier lifestyle, for a long, healthy, happy life.

Patricia herself is the symbol of health, perpetual youthfulness & natural femininity, radiant & super energy. She is a living & sparkling example of her & her father's healthy lifestyle precepts & this she loves sharing world-wide.

A fifth-generation Californian on her mother's side, Patricia was reared by The Bragg Natural Health Method from infancy. In school, she not only excelled in athletics, she won honors for her studies & counseling. She is an accomplished musician & dancer, tennis player & mountain climber. Patricia is a popular gifted Health Teacher, a dynamic personality & perfect Talk Show Guest on Radio & TV Shows where she regularly spreads the simple, easy-to-follow Bragg Healthy Lifestyle for everyone of all ages. Patricia's been on the covers of many magazines as her health message is needed & well received by millions.

Man's body is his vehicle through life, his earthly temple & the Creator wants us filled with joy & health for a long, fulfilled life. The Bragg Crusades of Health & Fitness (3 John 2) has carried her around the world over 30 times – spreading physical, emotional, mental & spiritual health & joy. Health is our birthright & Patricia teaches how to prevent the destruction of our health from man-made wrong lifestyle habits of living.

Patricia's been a Health Consultant to American Presidents, British Royalty, to Champion Triathletes *(She wrote 600 page Tri-Health Fitness Manual)*, Betty Cuthbert, Australia's "Golden Girl" (16 world records & 4 Olympic track gold medals), & New Zealand's Olympic Track & Triathlete Star, Allison Roe. Among those who follow her advice are some of Hollywood's top Stars from Clint Eastwood to ever-youthful singing group – The Beach Boys, Singing Stars of Metropolitan Opera & top Ballet Stars, etc. Patricia's message is of world-wide appeal & well received by people of all ages, nationalities & walks-of-life. Those who follow The Bragg Healthy Lifestyle & attend The Bragg Crusades world-wide are living testimonials . . . like ageless, super athlete, Jack LaLanne, who at age 15 went from sickness to Total Fitness & Health!